Quantitative Electroencephalographic Analysis (QEEG) Databases for Neurotherapy: Description, Validation, and Application

Quantitative Electroencephalographic Analysis (QEEG) Databases for Neurotherapy: Description, Validation, and Application

Joel F. Lubar, PhD
Editor

informa

healthcare

New York   London

First published in 2003 by Haworth Medical Press, Inc.

This edition published in 2010 by Informa Healthcare, Telephone House, 69-77 Paul Street, London EC2A 4LQ, UK.

Simultaneously published in the USA by Informa Healthcare, 52 Vanderbilt Avenue, 7th Floor, New York, NY 10017, USA.

Informa Healthcare is a trading division of Informa UK Ltd. Registered Office: 37–41 Mortimer Street, London W1T 3JH, UK. Registered in England and Wales number 1072954.

A CIP record for this book is available from the British Library.

Library of Congress Cataloging-in-Publication Data available on application

ISBN-13: 9780789004888

Orders may be sent to: Informa Healthcare, Sheepen Place, Colchester, Essex CO3 3LP, UK
Telephone: +44 (0)20 7017 5540
Email: CSDhealthcarebooks@informa.com
Website: http://informahealthcarebooks.com/

For corporate sales please contact: CorporateBooksIHC@informa.com
For foreign rights please contact: RightsIHC@informa.com
For reprint permissions please contact: PermissionsIHC@informa.com
Printed and bound by CPI Group (UK) Ltd, Croydon, CR0 4YY
Transferred to Digital Print 2012

Quantitative Electroencephalographic Analysis (QEEG) Databases for Neurotherapy: Description, Validation, and Application

CONTENTS

Foreword   xiii
David L. Trudeau, MD

Preface   xv
Joel F. Lubar, PhD

SCIENTIFIC ARTICLES

Parametric and Non-Parametric Analysis of QEEG:
Normative Database Comparisons in Electroencephalography,
a Simulation Study on Accuracy   1
Marco Congedo, PhD
Joel F. Lubar, PhD

Use of Databases in QEEG Evaluation   31
Jack Johnstone, PhD
Jay Gunkelman, QEEG-D

Quantitative EEG Normative Databases: A Comparative
Investigation   53
Tamara D. Lorensen, BSc Grad Dip
Paul Dickson, BSocSc Bpsych

Databases or Specific Training Protocols for Neurotherapy?
A Proposal for a "Clinical Approach to Neurotherapy"   69
Jaime Romano-Micha, MD

Quantitative EEG Normative Databases: Validation
   and Clinical Correlation   87
      Robert W. Thatcher, PhD
      Rebecca A. Walker, BS
      Carl J. Biver, PhD
      Duane N. North, MS
      Richard Curtin, MA

Comparison of QEEG Reference Databases in Basic Signal
   Analysis and in the Evaluation of Adult ADHD   123
      J. Noland White, PhD

Index   171

ABOUT THE EDITOR

Joel F. Lubar, PhD, received his BS and PhD from the Division of Biological Sciences and the Department of Biopsychology at the University of Chicago. He is currently Full Professor at the University of Tennessee. Dr. Lubar has published more than 100 papers, wrote many book chapters and eight books in the area of neuroscience and applied psychophysiology. Dr. Lubar is Associate Editor for the *Journal of Neurotherapy*, and has been a Regional Editor for the journal *Physiology and Behavior*, Associate Editor for *Biofeedback and Self Regulation*, and a member of the Editorial Board for the journal of *Applied Psychophysiology and Biofeedback*. He is President-Elect of the International Society for Neuronal Regulation (ISNR), and has been Co-Director of Southeastern Biofeedback and Neurobehavioral Institute in Knoxville since 1979. Dr. Lubar was the first President of the Biofeedback Society of Tennessee, had been President of the Academy of Certified Neurotherapists, which he incorporated into the Biofeedback Certification Institute of America EEG Specialty area (BCIA-EEG), has been president of the EEG Division of the Association for Applied Psychophysiology and Biofeedback (AAPB) and was President of AAPB in 1996-1997.

In the mid-1970s, Dr. Lubar was responsible for developing the application of EEG biofeedback (neurofeedback) as a treatment modality for children, adolescents, and adults with attention deficit hyperactivity disorder. This application of neurofeedback is one of the largest and used in clinics and schools throughout the United States, Canada, and parts of South America, Europe, Israel, and China. Dr. Lubar has been involved in the development of databases for the assessment of individuals with ADD/HD and has been a scientific advisor for a number of organizations that are involved in developing research to validate this application of neurofeedback. He has presented his research in many workshops in Europe, Japan, Australia, Israel, South America, Canada and to many state and national meetings of biofeedback organizations. In 1992, he and his colleagues published a paper in *Pediatric Neurology* showing for the first time that children with the inattentive form of ADD without hyperactivity differed significantly in terms of quantitative EEG parameters from matched non-clinical controls. Dr. Lubar is currently involved in research using an inverse solution technique known as Low Resolution Electromagnetic Tomography (LORETA), which allows one to locate current source generators inside the cortex that are responsible for the surface distribution of EEG. He and his colleagues at the University of Tennessee are now attempting to train individuals using LORETA neurofeedback to change activity inside the brain. This is the first attempt to use the inverse solution for this application.

Foreword

This monograph on quantitative electroencephalographic (QEEG) databases was conceived by Dr. Joel Lubar, one of the outstanding pioneers of neurotherapy and an unquestioned leader in the field. The field of neurotherapy owes a special debt of gratitude to Dr. Lubar for coming up with the concept for this publication and for recruiting the authors of the important papers that it contains. I know that Dr. Lubar has spent many long hours reviewing and coordinating peer reviews for the papers that appear here. As editor, he has done an outstanding job of recruiting quality papers and seeing them through review and revision to this final product. The evolving science of QEEG databases is of interest to clinical neurobiofeedback, and also to the broad fields of neuro-electrophysiology and EEG neurology. This book will be available to neurophysiologists, neuropsychiatrists, neurologists, neuropsychologists and neurotherapists who are not regular subscribers to the *Journal of Neurotherapy* or members of the International Society for Neuronal Regulation (ISNR), and who otherwise would not be apprised of the progress in QEEG databases in clinical neurotherapy. The commentaries and research on QEEG databases in this collection are from a perspective of clinical neurotherapy. As such they are broad and far reaching, and it is hoped this volume will further the cross-fertilization of dialogues between neurotherapy clinicians and EEG neuroscientists.

Other monographs on clinical neurotherapy are currently in the planning and development stages. A collection on hemoencephalography is planned for publication in 2004. Hemoencephalography is concerned with brain blood flow, as measured by surface oximetry, or by infrared measurements, and is the basis for a novel neurotherapy finding application in biofeedback paradigms as a treatment for migraine headaches and other conditions. Tim Tinius, PhD, of the psychology department at St. Cloud State University in Minnesota will be the editor of this book. A publication is also in the planning stages for neurotherapy applications in educational settings, focussing on non-drug therapy approaches for attentional disorders and learning disabilities. Also, a volume is planned for neurotherapy applications in criminal justice settings, employing brain wave biofeedback strategies for addictive disorders and other problems frequently found in criminal justice populations. Advances in these three areas has been substantial and warrants publication in a convenient hard bound format available to students, teachers, clinicians and others interested in these topics. Also, these monographs offer an opportunity for clinicians and researchers in neurotherapy (the application of biofeedback and self modulation based on neurophysiology to clinical practice) the opportunity to make their work available to a wide readership.

David L. Trudeau, MD
Editor
Journal of Neurotherapy

Preface

DATABASES:
A GUIDE MAP TO PRECISION
FOR NEUROFEEDBACK PROTOCOLS, TRAINING
AND RESEARCH

I am very pleased to have had the opportunity to act as the editor for this monograph dedicated specifically to databases and to present this outstanding set of papers dealing with the development and validation of databases. I want to express my appreciation to David Trudeau, the Editor-in-Chief of the *Journal of Neurotherapy*, and to Darlene Nelson, Managing Editor of the *Journal*, for their considerable help working with me on this endeavor. For many of us in the field of neurotherapy, quantitative electroencephalographic (QEEG) databases are very important. For those of us who rely on databases for research and for clinical practice, they represent the cornerstone of the methodology necessary to help us in differentiating cognitive states, clinical disorders, and EEG changes throughout the lifespan.

The development and validation of databases has also been a very controversial area. In the 1990s there were papers published by the American Academy of Neurology and the American Clinical Neurophysiological Society criticizing the use of quantitative EEG based on digital analysis. Hoffman et al. (1999) represented a response in which all of the earlier criticisms were described and put forth a significant rebuttal. Since that time there have not been any significant published criticisms of databases similar to those that appeared before our response. This indicates that as of the summer of 1999 significant progress had been made in the development, validation, and use of databases in the evaluation of traumatic brain injury, attention deficit disorders, learning disabilities, seizure disorders, depression, anxiety disorders, and perhaps additional neurological and neuropsychiatric disorders. Adam Clarke and R. Barry's group in Australia have published 13 papers since 1998, most during the years 2001 and 2002 and some during the current year, showing the effectiveness of quantitative EEG for evaluation of attention deficit disorder, oppositional defiant disorder, reading disabilities, and the differentiation of these from other behavioral disorders (see References).

Though significant recent progress has been made in the development of databases there are still numerous problems dealing with the limitation of databases to primarily eyes-open, eyes-closed or relatively few cognitive tasks. There are problems related to selection of non-clinical controls and their screening as well as selection criteria for individuals experiencing different clinical disorders. Databases still must be improved in terms of the number of subjects for different age groups, criteria for artifact rejection, selection of band passes for data collection and cross validation for different multi-channel EEG instruments.

The papers in this volume were developed by people who have had considerable experience in either the development of databases or in working with them. They point out strengths, limitations, and provide in some cases, comparative information for the different databases that are currently in use. It is hoped that the information contained in this collection will provide a foundation for people who are interested in using databases and particularly for the future development of better databases which will include both eyes-open and eyes-closed as well as numerous cognitive tasks with large numbers of cases both clinical and non-clinical in each age group. I can say clearly from my own personal experience having worked with well over 2,000 patients with attentional problems as well as other disorders during the past 25 years that with the development of databases my own ability to fine tune existing protocols and develop new protocols for neurotherapy has been greatly improved, leading to better treatment, better long term outcome, and fewer training sessions. For me, quantitative EEG with a good database is a road map that clearly points the direction for the development of treatment paradigms. Many others in our field have experienced the same benefits. In this context, I emphasize that when we speak of quantitative EEG this does not necessarily mean 19 channels; it can be one channel to 19 or even more. At the present time there are no databases for 24, 32 or more channels. Perhaps those will be developed in the future but at the present time the standard 19-channel data collection with appropriate use of existing databases can lead to very accurate and outstanding clinical results.

Joel F. Lubar, PhD
Editor

REFERENCES

Barry, R., Clarke, A., McCarthy, R., & Selikowitz, M. (2002). EEG coherence in attention-deficit/hyperactivity disorder: A comparative study of two DSM-IV types. *Clinical Neurophysiology, 113*, 579-585.

Barry, R. J., Johnstone, S. J., Clarke, A. R. (2003). A review of electrophysiology in attention-deficit/hyperactivity disorder: II. Event-related potentials. *Clinical Neurophysiology, 114*, 184-198.

Barry, R., Kirkaikul, S., & Hodder, D. (2000). EEG alpha activity and the ERP to target stimuli in an auditory oddball paradigm. *International Journal of Psychophysiology, 39*, 39-50.

Clarke, A., Barry, R., McCarthy, R., & Selikowitz, M. (1998). EEG analysis in attention-deficit/hyperactivity disorder: A comparative study of two subtypes. *Psychiatry Research, 81*, 19-29.

Clarke, A., Barry, R., McCarthy, R., & Selikowitz, M. (2001). Age and sex effects in the EEG: Differences in two subtypes of attention-deficit/hyperactivity disorder. *Clinical Neurophysiology, 112*, 806-814.

Clarke, A., Barry, R., McCarthy, R., & Selikowitz, M. (2001). Age and sex effects in the EEG: Development of the normal child. *Clinical Neurophysiology, 112*, 815-826.

Clarke, A., Barry, R., McCarthy, R., & Selikowitz, M. (2001). EEG-defined subtypes of children with attention-deficit/hyperactivity disorder. *Clinical Neurophysiology, 112*, 2098-2105.

Clarke, A., Barry, R., McCarthy, R., & Selikowitz, M. (2001). Excess beta in children with attention-deficit/hyperactivity disorder: An atypical electrophysiological group. *Psychiatry Research, 103*, 205-218.

Clarke, A., Barry, R., McCarthy, R., & Selikowitz, M. (2001). EEG differences in two subtypes of children with attention-deficit/hyperactivity disorder. *Psychophysiology, 38*, 212-221.

Clarke, A., Barry, R., McCarthy, R., & Selikowitz, M. (2002). Children with attention-deficit/hyperactivity disorder and comorbid oppositional defiant disorder: An EEG analysis. *Psychiatry Research, 111*, 181-190.

Clarke, A., Barry, R., McCarthy, R., & Selikowitz, M. (2002). EEG analysis of children with attention-deficit/hyperactivity disorder and comorbid reading disabilities. *Journal of Learning Disabilities, 35*, 276-285.

Clarke, A., Barry, R., McCarthy, R., Selikowitz, M., & Brown, C. R. (2002). EEG evidence for a new conceptualization of attention-deficit/hyperactivity disorder. *Clinical Neurophysiology, 113*, 1-36.

Clarke, A., Barry, R., McCarthy, R., & Selikowitz, M. (2003). Hyperkinetic disorder in the ICD-10: EEG evidence for a definitional widening? *European Child and Adolescent Psychiatry*, *12*, 92-99.

Hoffman, D. A., Lubar, J. F., Thatcher, R. W., Sterman, M. B., Rosenfeld, P. J., Striefel, S., et al. (1999). Limitations of the American Academy of Neurology and American Clinical Neurophysiology Society paper on QEEG. *Journal of Neuropsychiatry Clinical Neuroscience*, *11*, 401-407.

SCIENTIFIC ARTICLES

Parametric and Non-Parametric Analysis of QEEG: Normative Database Comparisons in Electroencephalography, a Simulation Study on Accuracy

Marco Congedo, PhD
Joel F. Lubar, PhD

SUMMARY. Quantitative electroencephalography (QEEG) as a tool for the diagnosis of neurological and psychiatric disorders is receiving

Marco Congedo is affiliated with, and Joel F. Lubar is Professor, Department of Psychology, Brain Research and Psychophysiology Laboratory, The University of Tennessee, Knoxville, TN.

Address correspondence to: Joel F. Lubar, PhD, Department of Psychology, 310 Austin Peay Building, University of Tennessee, Knoxville, TN 37996-0900 (E-mail: jlubar@utk.edu).

The authors want to express their gratitude to Dr. Robert Pascual-Marqui, whose work greatly influenced this study, and whose comments gave the first author the idea underlying this article. The authors are also grateful to Leslie Sherlin, who patiently corrected the original manuscript.

increased interest. While QEEG analysis is restricted to the scalp, the recent development of electromagnetic tomography (ET) allows the study of the electrical activity of all cortical structures. Electrical measures from a patient can be compared with a normative database derived from a large sample of healthy individuals. The deviance from the database norms provides a measure of the likelihood that the patient's electrical activity reflects abnormal brain functioning. The focus of this article is a method for estimating such deviance. The traditional method based on z-scores (parametric) is reviewed and a new method based on percentiles (non-parametric) is proposed. The parametric and the non-parametric methods are compared using simulated data. The accuracy of both methods is assessed as a function of normative sample size and gaussianity for three different alpha levels. Results suggest that the performance of the parametric method is unaffected by sample size, given that the sample size is large enough (N > 100), but that non-gaussianity jeopardizes accuracy even if the normative distribution is close to gaussianity. In contrast, the performance of the non-parametric method is unaffected by non-gaussianity, but is a function of sample size only. It is shown that with N > 160, the non-parametric method is always preferable. Results will be discussed taking into consideration technical issues related to the nature of QEEG and ET data. It will be suggested that the sample size is the only constant across EEG frequency bands, measurement locations, and kind of quantitative measures. As a consequence, for a given database, the error rate of the non-parametric database is homogeneous; however, the same is not true for the parametric method. *[Article copies available for a fee from The Haworth Document Delivery Service: 1-800-HAWORTH. E-mail address: <docdelivery@haworthpress.com> Website: <http://www.HaworthPress. com> © 2003 by The Haworth Press, Inc. All rights reserved.]*

KEYWORDS. EEG, QEEG, quantitative electroencephalography, normative database, norms, non-parametric

INTRODUCTION

Comparison to quantitative electroencephalography (QEEG) norms is a valuable tool in both electrophysiological research and clinical practice. Typically, the individual's electroencephalogram is analyzed in the frequency domain by means of time series analysis techniques such as the Fast Fourier Transform, also called FFT (Beauchamp, 1973; Brillinger, 1975; Lynn & Fuerst, 1989). A certain number of features are extracted from the Fourier cross-spectral matrix, each one describing a particular feature of the brainwaves in a specified frequency range.

These may include univariate and multivariate measures of absolute power, relative power and mean frequency for each electrode location in addition to coherence, phase and asymmetry for each electrode pair. Each individual's quantitative feature is called a *descriptor*. Descriptors are compared to norms derived under the same conditions from a sample of healthy "normal" subjects, allowing the statistical estimation of the deviance from the population norms. A recent trend in the electrophysiological literature is the derivation of norms for electromagnetic tomographic data (Bosch-Bayard et al., 2001). Electromagnetic tomographies (ET) make use of the EEG potential difference recording on the scalp to estimate the current density within the brain. Functional images of the current density distribution are then superimposed onto MRI standard atlas anatomical images (Talairach & Tournoux, 1988), providing true neuroimaging of electromagnetic brain activity either in the time or in the frequency domain. The most popular ET is the Low Resolution Electromagnetic Tomography, better known as LORETA (Fuchs, Wagner, Kohler, & Wischmann, 1999; Pascual-Marqui, 1995, 1999; Pascual-Marqui, Michel, & Lehmann, 1994). The derivation of norms for current density data is analogous to the derivation of norms for QEEG. In the former, electrical activity is not measured on the scalp at the electrode level, but estimated within the brain in discrete cubic regions of arbitrary size called voxels. Since, typically, one defines thousands of voxels, but makes use of only 19 to 128 electrodes, the comparison to ET norms poses more stringent statistical problems than the comparison to the QEEG norms. In both cases the deviance from each norm is usually expressed in terms of z-scores. The method assumes gaussianity of the sampling distribution and hereafter will be referred to as "parametric." The assumption of gaussianity is not always matched with real data. The aim of this article is to propose an equivalent "non-parametric" method based on percentiles for the estimation of the deviance from the norms. Furthermore, by means of a simulation we compared the two methods in terms of accuracy. The non-parametric method applies equally well to QEEG and to ET data.

The Nature of EEG

It is clear that in utilizing EEG norms we make several assumptions regarding the nature of human EEG. Essentially we assume that the human EEG is a stationary process with relatively high intra-subjects and inter-subjects reliability. Those assumptions are critical for the validity of the comparison process. Most of the initial work in this respect has been done by E. Roy John and his associates (Ahn et al., 1980; John et al., 1977, 1980a, 1980b; John, Prichep, Fridman, & Easton, 1988). First, it was shown that quantitative EEG measures follow developmental equations, meaning that the frequency composition of the EEG reflects the age and the functional status of the brain. In other words, in a normal condition, normal values depend on and can be predicted by age (Ahn et al., 1980; John et al., 1980a, 1980b; Gasser, Verleger, Bacher, & Stroka, 1988; Matthis, Scheffner, Benninger, Lipinsky, & Stolzis, 1980). For example, the relationship may be quadratic on the log of the age. This is the case of the dominant frequency power of the normal EEG, which increases during brain development and declines slowly after age thirty or so (Bosch-Bayard et al., 2001; John, Prichep, & Easton, 1987; Szava et al., 1994). As a result, data from a wide age-range database is modeled by means of polynomial regression equations in order to take into account the age differences (John et al., 1980a, 1980b). There is little evidence suggesting that EEG norms may vary significantly as a function of sex and hemispheric dominance (Matthis et al., 1980; Veldhuizen, Jonkman, & Poortvliet, 1993). If such effects are found in the data, corrections for these two factors should be applied as well. Second, it is well known that the intra-subject spectral descriptors of the EEG are consistent over short periods of time, probably as a result of stable homeostatic regulations of the neurotransmitters (Hughes & John, 1999). This is particularly true for the EEG recorded during a resting state where the subjects have their eyes closed, and for relative power measures (John et al., 1987). Another advantage of relative measures is that they are independent of factors such as skin and skull thickness, being invariant in respect to a global scale power factor that increases inter-subjects variability (Hernández et al., 1994). For these reasons QEEG normative databases are usually generated for the eyes-closed resting state only, and relative power measures are preferred. Third, normative QEEG descriptors were found to be independent from cultural and ethnic factors. High reliability was found in studies from Barbados, China, Cuba, Germany, Holland, Japan, Korea, Mexico, Netherlands, Sweden, the United States, and Venezuela (quoted and referenced in Hughes & John, 1999).

The independence of the EEG spectrum from cultural and ethnic factors is a remarkable characteristic of the EEG. It has been suggested that it reflects the common genetic heritage of mankind (Hughes & John, 1999). A study on a large sample of 16-year-old twins found that the variance of EEG power (76% to 89% depending on the frequency band) is mostly explained by heritability (van Beijsterveldt, Molenaar, de Gaus, & Boosma, 1996). The authors conclude that the EEG frequency pattern is one of the most heritable characteristics in humans. Fourth,

QEEG norms proved to have high specificity and sensitivity. When subjects with no neurological or psychiatric dysfunction are compared with norms, only a few descriptors show significant deviance (high specificity). On the contrary, when subjects with neurological or psychiatric dysfunctions are compared to norms, the number of significant deviant descriptors greatly exceeds the number expected by chance alone (high sensitivity; John, Prichep, Fridman, & Easton, 1988).

Comparisons to QEEG norms has proven useful in the diagnosis of the attention deficit disorder with and without hyperactivity, learning disabilities, dementia, schizophrenia, unipolar and bipolar depression, anxiety disorders, obsessive-compulsive disorder, alcohol and substance abuse, head injury, lesions, tumors, epilepsy, and cerebrovascular diseases. (For a review see Hughes & John, 1999; Nuwer, 1988.) For many other disorders and diseases, QEEG signatures have been found, but additional research is needed to establish usefulness for diagnostic purposes. The four characteristics of the EEG power spectrum mentioned previously can be considered the fundamental properties of QEEG since they enable objective assessment of brain integrity in persons of any age, origin or background.

Signal Detection Theory and Diagnostic Systems

In this section we briefly review some important concepts in the literature on signal detection theory. These concepts will provide us with a workable framework to compare the parametric and non-parametric methods. Normative databases are essentially diagnostic systems. The general task of diagnostic systems is to discriminate among possible states of the object under study, and to decide which one actually exists. In the case of normative databases, the task is to label the descriptor of the new individual as "normal" or "abnormal," or, using a more appropriate terminology, as "non-deviant" or "deviant." No diagnostic system is perfectly accurate. Modern detection theory treats the decision in probabilistic terms, according to which there are two statistical hypotheses. In the following discussion we will refer to a particular descriptor only. The arguments readily extend to an indeterminate number of descriptors.

The study of the accuracy of diagnostic systems sprang from signal detection theory and is a common subject in the biomedical literature (Swets, 1988; Swets & Pickett, 1982). In comparing to norms the system receives an input, the value of the descriptor, and makes one of two possible decisions. We will refer to the input, or actual status of the new individual, as the "event" (E). E can take on two mutually exclusive values. Let us label them as positive (+) or negative (−) which we will use hereafter instead of "deviant" and "non-deviant," respectively. E+ is the event corresponding to a true deviance from the norms, and E− is the event corresponding to a true non-deviance from the norms. Notice that the status of the subject is given and not observed. The system output is the decision taken. We will refer to this output based on the decision of the database and call it "diagnosis" (D). D can also take on two mutually exclusive values. Following the same notation we will have D+ in the case of a positive decision (the new individual is decided to be deviant) and D− in the case of a negative decision (the new individual is decided to be non-deviant). With two alternative events and two corresponding diagnosis, the data of a test of accuracy is conveniently summarized in a two-by-two contingency table (Table 1). We wish to obtain perfect correspondence between the events and the diagnosis. That is, we wish that the value of the descriptor for a new subject is labeled as deviant if it is in reality deviant and non-deviant if it is in reality non-deviant. These two outcomes correspond to the agreement (or concordance) between the input and the output of the diagnostic system, referred to in Table 1 as true positive (TP) and true negative (TN). When there is no agreement then we have an error, which can be of two types: false positive (FP) and false negative (FN). If we consider proportions instead of raw frequencies of the four outcomes, then just two proportions contain all of the information about the observed outcomes (Swets, 1988). For instance we normalize each raw frequency in a cell by the column total. We have now:

$$TP = TP/(TP + FN); \; FN = FN/(TP + FN); \; FP = FP/(FP + TN);$$
$$TN = TN/(FP + TN)$$

In this way we obtain proportion estimations (analogous to probability values) bounded between zero and one and the following properties hold:

$$TP + FN = 1; \; FP + N = 1$$

In other words, the elements of the couples TP-FN and FP-TN are complements of each other and all the information about the observed outcomes can be obtained considering only one element for each couple. Furthermore, by normalizing the raw frequencies we obtain measures *independent of the prior probability of the event*, meaning that the estimation of errors will be independent of the proportions of positive events (E+) and negative events (E−) entered in the system (Swets, 1988). This is a fundamental property of any accuracy measure of diagnostic system. Figure 1 shows these normalized measures in a different, albeit equivalent, perspective. Organizing the same data in a probability tree diagram we see that what we are computing, equivalently, are the probabilities to have positive or negative diagnosis (D+ and D−) *conditional* on the probability that the event was positive or negative (E+ and E−). For example, the rate of normalized true positives is the probability to have a positive diagnosis given (conditional on the fact) that the event was positive. In notation we write p(E+|D+). This quantity (normalized TP) is also referred to as 'sensitivity' (SN) and is usually reported together with the normalized TN, or p(E−|D−), which is referred to as "specificity" (SP). SN is a measure of the ability of the system to take a positive decision when it is indeed the case. Its complement is the normalized FN proportion. The SP is a measure of the ability of the system to take a negative decision when it is indeed the case. Its complement is the normalized FP proportion. According to what we have said before, SN and SP summarize the contingency table exhaustively.

TABLE 1

		Event (E)	[Input]
		Positive	Negative
Diagnosis (D)	Positive	TRUE POSITIVE	FALSE POSITIVE
[Output]	Negative	FALSE NEGATIVE	TRUE NEGATIVE

FIGURE 1. Probability Tree. The same data summarized in Table 1 can be arranged, after normalization, in a probability tree. The tree shows the resulting conditional probabilities. See text for details.

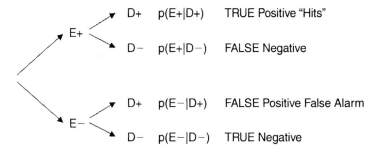

	D+	p(E+	D+)	TRUE Positive "Hits"
E+	D−	p(E+	D−)	FALSE Negative
E−	D+	p(E−	D+)	FALSE Positive False Alarm
	D−	p(E−	D−)	TRUE Negative

However, for the purpose of our simulation, a more complete depiction of the errors committed by a normative database is achieved considering two additional measures. These are the *inverse probability* of a true positive response and the inverse probability of a true negative response (Guggenmoos-Holzmann & Houwelingen, 2000; Swets & Pickett, 1982).

Practically, what we want to know is the probability that a deviance exists when the system says it does, and the probability that a deviance does not exist when the system says it does not. These definitions are not just a play on the words (see previous definitions of SN and SP). We seek p(E+|D+) and p(E−|D−), respectively, the *inverse* probability of SN and SP (to obtain those you need to invert the position of E and D). These probabilities are easily computed arranging the data as in Figure 1 and using the formula defining the conditional probability or the Bayes' formula (Lipschutz & Lipson, 2000). The agreement E+D+ corresponds to the true acceptance of the alternative hypotheses "the new individual is deviant on that descriptor," while the agreement E−D− corresponds to the true rejection of this alternative hypotheses. Accordingly, we will refer to the quantity p(E+|D+) as "true acceptance" (TA) and to the quantity p(E−|D−) as "true rejection" (TR). For reasons that will be clear later, only considering together SN, SP, TA, and TR, will enable us to perform a complete and fair estimation of the systematic error rate for the parametric and non-parametric methods.

The Parametric Method Based on Z-Scores

We are now ready to turn to the issue of deviance estimation. The steps required in order to build a normative database according to the parametric method (PM) and to the non-parametric method (nPM) are listed in Table 2. The focus of this article is steps 5 and 7 in Table 2, and in fact, these are the only two steps where the procedures for the PM and the nPM differ. We are concerned here with the way in which the significance of the deviance is estimated. We will not discuss the sampling of the normative subjects (which determine the homogeneity and representativeness of the normative sample) or the issue of multiple comparisons (which is essential to avoid false positives). Based on our review of the literature, all published normative EEG and QEEG databases estimated the significance of the deviance according to a parametric method based on z-scores (e.g., Bosch-Bayard et al., 2001; John et al., 1987; Thatcher, 1999; Veldhuizen et al., 1993). The work of John and his colleagues was decisive for the development and assessment of this statistical methodology (John et al., 1977). When z-scores at each electrode location are interpolated to construct brain topographical maps, the result is called "Significance Probability Mapping," or SPM (Duffy, Bartels, & Burchfiel, 1981). In step 3 of Table 2 we defined the descriptors of our own LORETA database. According to the notation used in Table 2, there are d = L × F descriptors for each normative subject (i.e., for each subject there is a descriptor) for each combination of location (electrode for QEEG and voxel for ET) and feature (quantitative measure in a specified frequency range). For example, a descriptor is the relative power in the alpha range, and another descriptor is the relative power in the theta range. Thus, each descriptor can be conceived as a vector comprised of N values, where N is the number of subjects in the database. Let us call x_d the vectors of the descriptor d. For each feature, the appropriate log-transformation is applied to all subjects (John et al., 1987). The resulting data distribution of the vectors x_d is approximately normal with mean y_d and standard deviation σ_d. In step 6 we considered the L × F matrix of descriptors referring to a new individual to be compared to the database. Notice that the L × F matrix for the normative database is a matrix of vectors (i.e., a 3-D matrix). Instead for any new individual the L × F matrix is a 2-D matrix of individual entries. Identical log-transformations are applied to this matrix as well. Let us call $\hat{y}_d$ each entry of the descriptor matrix for the new individual. The task is to obtain an estimation of the deviance, from the mean of the x_d, for each $\hat{y}_d$. Given gaussianity of the normative sample distribution, the deviance of the new individual for each descriptor d is estimated as

$$z_d = (\hat{y}_d - y_d)/\sigma_d \ [1.0]$$

The mean of the normative sample is subtracted from the new individual's descriptor and the result is divided by the standard deviation of the normative sample. The z-scores computed with 1.0 are accurate if the normative sample distribution is normal (gaussian). The more the normative sample distribution deviates from normality, the less the z-scores will be accurate, leading to more and more false negatives and false positives as a function of the distribution skewness and kurtosis. Skewness refers to the third moment around the mean of a distribution and is a measure of asymmetry. For example, a chi-square distribution with one degree of freedom is said to be right-skewed. Kurtosis is the fourth moment around the mean and is a measure of the peakedness of the distribution. A "flat" distribution has higher kurtosis than a "peaked" one. A theoretical standard normal distribution has skewness = 0 and

TABLE 2

Steps	Parametric Method	Non-Parametric Method
1	A reference Population (usually normal) is defined and a sample of **N** subjects is selected. Each subject is screened in order to match inclusion criteria previously chosen. The **N** subjects constitute the database.	A reference Population (usually normal) is defined and a sample of **N** subjects is selected. Each subject is screened in order to match inclusion criteria previously chosen. The **N** subjects constitute the database.
2	The set of **F** features is defined. Each feature refers to a quantitative measure for a particular frequency range. For example, a feature could be "Delta Relative Power" or "Alpha Coherence."	The set of **F** features is defined. Each feature refers to a quantitative measure for a particular frequency range. For example, a feature could be "Delta Relative Power" or "Alpha Coherence."
3	For each of the **N** subjects constituting the database, for each location (electrode or voxel) or pair of locations (electrodes or voxels), **L** measures for each of the chosen set of **F** features are derived. Each combination of measure and feature is called **Descriptor**.	For each of the **N** subjects constituting the database, for each location (electrode or voxel) or pair of locations (electrodes or voxels), **L** measures for each of the chosen set of **F** features are derived. Each combination of measure and feature is called **Descriptor**.
4	Database Data form a $L \times F \times N$ matrix.	Database Data form a $L \times F \times N$ matrix.
5	For each feature, an appropriate transformation (based on log) is applied to all locations and subjects in order to approximate gaussianity.	For each feature and location the **N** data of the database subjects is sorted.
6	For each new individual to be compared to the database, a corresponding data matrix of descriptors ($L \times F$) is derived.	For each new individual to be compared to the database, a corresponding data matrix of descriptors ($L \times F$) is derived.
7	For each location (**L**) and feature (**F**), i.e., for each descriptor, the deviation from normality is expressed in terms of z-scores, using the mean and standard deviation of the descriptor computed for all database subjects.	For each location (**L**) and feature (**F**), i.e., for each descriptor, the deviation from normality is expressed in terms of discrete random variable sp (sample proportion) expressing the proportion of the subjects in the database falling above (right-handed test) or below (left-handed test) the new individual.
8	Additional statistics are performed in order to correct for multiple comparisons.	Additional statistics are performed in order to correct for multiple comparisons.

kurtosis = 3. Given an approximate gaussian distribution, the more these two values deviate from the theoretical values, the more the distribution deviates from gaussianity. The problem with the rate of false positives and false negatives in the case of non-gaussian distributions is a subtle one. With estimation [1.0] we obtain different rates of false positives and false negatives depending on the side of skewness (left-skewed or right-skewed distribution) and the side of the test (left-handed or right-handed test). Similar arguments apply to the amount of kurtosis.

The effects of skewness and kurtosis on the rate of false positives and false negatives are easily captured in a graphical fashion (Figure 2). This figure is crucial for the interpretation of the results of this study and should be analyzed carefully by the reader. Figure 2a depicts a normative sampling distribution very close to the theoretical gaussian. Suppose that distribution is indeed gaussian. With an alpha level of 0.05, the decision criterion of the database is to label as "deviant" all new observations with z-score > 1.96 or < -1.96 (the area under the curve for $z > 1.96$ or $z < -1.96$ equals 0.025, so their sum is 0.05). Let us consider the right-handed test first. A z-score exceeding 1.96 leaves on its right a proportion of the area under the curve less than 0.025. So the diagnosis will be positive (D+). By definition, a new individual's score with $p < 0.025$ is positive (E+). The result is a concordance between the event and the diagnosis (true positive).

Because of simmetricity, for a left-handed test the result will be the same. For all z-scores comprised between -1.96 and 1.96 both the event and the diagnosis will be negative (E− and D−), and we will have concordance again (true negative). Thus if the normative sampling distribution is truly gaussian, the normative database will virtually commit no error. Figure 2b depicts a normative sampling distribution right skewed. Notice that the mean of the distribution (blue line) is no longer at the peak of the distribution since the density on the right side of the distribution is bigger than the density on the left side. The two violet vertical lines delimitate the interval including 95% of the density (area under the curve). On the right of the right violet line the density is 0.025%, and so it is on the left of the left violet line. Let us consider the right-handed test first. Because of skewness for a value of z slightly bigger than 1.96 (D+), the area under the curve on the right of the z-value is greater than 0.025 (E−). The diagnosis is positive ($z > 1.96$), but the event was not (area > 0.025). We have a false positive. In the hypothetical distribution of Figure 2b, the right-sided z-interval for which a false positive will happen is indicated in green. For the left-sided test the situation is opposite. Here for some $z > -1.96$ (D−) the area under the curve is already less than 0.025 (E+). The diagnosis is not positive, but the event was indeed positive. We obtain a false negative. In Figure 2b, the left-sided z interval for which a false negative will happen is, again, indicated in green. If the distribution is left-skewed, we would have obtained "mirror results" (i.e., false negatives on the right side of the dis-

FIGURE 2. Depiction of gaussian and non-gaussian distributions and the outcome of the parametric method. (a): The normality case. If the sample is truly gaussian then the outcome of the parametric normative database leads to true positives and true negatives only. (b) The non-normality case. The sample distribution is right skewed. On the right side of the distribution we have false positives, while on the left-side of the distribution we have false negative.

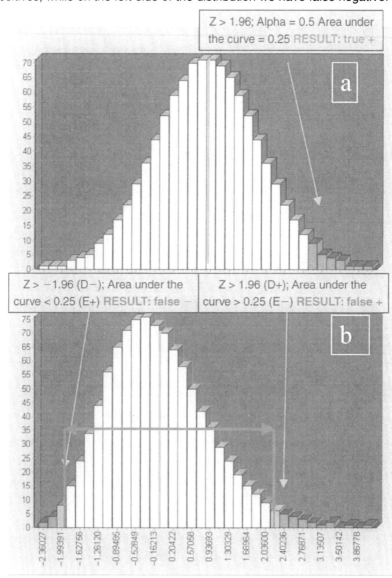

tributions and false positives on the left side). It is clear that with skewed normative sample distributions we obtain different types of errors on the two sides of the distribution. This means that what in reality are equivalent, but opposite, magnitude of deviances, are interpreted by the diagnostic system differently, according to the sign of the z-score. If the amount of error generated is not negligible, this property of the parametric method would constitute a serious problem. Therefore we need to estimate it. This will be accomplished in the simulation we are going to present. Before that, let us introduce an alternative method for the estimation of the deviance, a non-parametric method based on proportions.

The Non-Parametric Method Based on Proportions

In the previous section we have seen that the parametric method relies on the assumption of normality of the distribution. As a practical example, in a one-sided (right) testing framework, a z-score = 1.645 means that on the theoretical normal distribution 95% of the population falls below that value. In other words, only 5% of the population exhibits a value equal or greater. The corresponding value on the other side of the distribution (left-sided test) is -1.645, for which only 5% of the population exhibits a value equal or smaller. A non-parametric method, to obtain a similar result, is by use of the sample proportion (sp; Lunneborg, 1999). Sample proportions are analogous to percentiles and, like them, are obtained by sorting the sampling distribution values. The method is easily illustrated with an example. Refer first to a *right-handed test* with alpha = 0.05. In this case we label a new individual as deviant if his/her value is large as compared to the normative database. For example, if the descriptor under analysis is the alpha relative power at the electrode O2, then a deviant subject will show a large power value as compared to the norm. Suppose our normative sample is comprised of 20 subjects (N = 20). Let us sort the normative values referring to any descriptor d in ascending order to obtain the sorted x_d vector:

$$x_d: \{2, 2.5, 2.8, 3.5, 3.6, 3.7, 4, 4.9, 5.2, 5.7, 8.4, 8.5, 11.1, 12.3, 14.8, 16.4, 18.9, 20, 21, 25.4\}$$

The 95th percentile is the value below which 95% of the subjects fall. Values comprised between 21 and 25.4, leave on the right-side 5% of the observations (5% of 20 = 1). A value bigger than 21 is associated with a p-value < 0.05. We obtain a p-value with a counting random variable (e.g., Holmes, Blair, Watson & Ford, 1996). Let us define the discrete random variable (RV), sample proportion (Φ) as the *proportion of values in the x_d vector falling above the new individual's value*. Then Φ is indeed a p-value, although it is discrete and not continuous. By definition, if no value in the x_d vector exceeds the new individual's value, then $\Phi = 0$. In this case in fact the new individual shows the most extreme value and this is as significant (unlike) as it can possibly be. With this definition the discrete RV Φ can take on N+1 values ranging from 0 to 1 and decreasing by multiples of 1/n. $\Phi = 1$ (20/20 = 1) means that all normative subjects exceed the new individual's value. In this case the new individual's value is the smallest and there is no evidence at all that the new individual's value is significant (keep in mind that if our test is right-handed we have to ignore the extreme values on the left of the distribution, no matter how extreme they are). $\Phi = 0$ means that the new individual exhibits the most extreme value.

Suppose our new individual's value for the descriptor *d* is 22.3. Comparing this value to the sorted vector above we see that 5% of the observations fall above this value, thus Φ is 0.05 (there is only 1 observation falling above the value 22.3; 1/20 = 0.05). Suppose the value is 1.8; Φ is 1 (20/20 = 1). Suppose it is 5.4; Φ is 0.55 (11/20). $\Phi = 0.05$ can be considered deviant just like a z-score = 1.645. Both correspond to a probability of 0.05, with the difference that in a non-parametric fashion the p-value is computed on the actual data and not as a result of the integrals of the theoretical normal distribution.

The same method, reversed, is applied in the case of a *left-handed test*. In this case the discrete random variable (RV) sample proportion (Φ) is defined as the *proportion of values in the x_d vector falling below the new individual's value*. By definition, if all values in the x_d vector are bigger than the new individual's value, then $\Phi = 0$. In this case the new individual's value is the smallest and this provides the strongest evidence for his/her deviance on the left side of the distribution. With this reversed definition the discrete RV Φ still can take on N+1 values ranging form 0 to 1 and increasing by multiples of 1/n. $\Phi = 0$ means that all normative subjects exceed the new individual's value. $\Phi = 1$ means that the new individual's value exceed all normative subjects. Suppose again our new individual's value for the descriptor *d* is 22.3. For a left-handed test, comparing this value to the sorted vector above we see that 95% of the observations fall below this value, thus Φ is 0.95 (there are 19 observation falling below the value 22.3; 19/20 = 0.95). Suppose the value is 1.8; Φ is, by definition, 0. Suppose it is 5.4; Φ is 0.45 (9/20).

If a two-tailed test is wished, then the median of the distribution is computed. If the new individual's value is on the right of the median then a right-handed test as described is performed. On the other hand, if the new individual's value is on the left of the median then a left-handed test is performed. Of course, for a two-tailed test we need to halve the alpha level at the two sides of the distribution, so that the total alpha level equals indeed alpha. The performance of the non-parametric method here described is not affected by non-gaussianity of the sampling distribution. However its performance is a function of the sample size. Considering sample proportions we define a discrete RV, but the underlying phenomenon is continuous, hence we lose "resolution." In the following simulation we assess the amount of errors generated because of this loss of resolution and we compare it with the amount of error generated by the parametric method because of non-gaussianity.

METHOD

Simulation Study

In order to perform a simulation aiming to evaluate the performance of a normative database we need to define uniquely positive events (E+) and negative events (E−) (i.e., we need to delineate conditions under which a simulation entry is by definition deviant or non-deviant). Any particular method to make a decision about the deviance of the event will provide a diagnosis, either positive (D+) or negative (D−) according to its own procedure, and being unaware of the real status of the event. The agreement, or concordance, between the event and the diagnosis can then be estimated. By allowing a large number of events to enter the system we obtain reliable estimations of concordance and discordance. In order to define unambiguous positive and negative events we need to refer to theoretical distributions for which the "true" acceptance interval of the null hypothesis is known. For instance, let us set the type I error (alpha) as 0.05. For a random variable z distributed as a standard normal we accept the null hypothesis for $-1.96 < z < 1.96$. In other words, if z is comprised between -1.96 and 1.96, we accept the null hypothesis. In terms of a normative database this means that the new individual is considered to be normal. In our simulations the normative sample of reference was emulated by means of normal distributions. New individuals were emulated as individual points generated with the same density function as the normative reference. For all practical purposes they constitute events for which the status (E+ or E−) is known a priori on the basis of the distribution of the normative reference.

In the discussion that follows we will call each event submitted to diagnosis a *simulation entry*. As an example of the procedure followed to define simulation entries consider the following: given a normative reference sample distributed as a random normal, alpha = 0.05, and a right handed test, we know a priori that any simulation entry with p(z) < 0.025 is positive. For each simulation entry, we computed the database outcome (D+ or D−) with both the parametric and non-parametric method, independently one from the other. According to what is seen above, the parametric diagnosis is based on equation [1.0], and the non-parametric diagnosis is based on the RV sample proportion. For each simulation entry there will be a concordant or discordant outcome and this will add a raw frequency in a table just like Table 1. This constitutes an outcome among four possibilities (Table 1).

We submitted 100,000 simulation entries, under identical conditions, for each normative reference sample considered. This allowed reliable estimations of sensitivity (SN), specificity (SP), true acceptance (TA) and true rejection (TR). The evaluation of concordance was repeated varying sample size and gaussianity of the normative reference sample. This way we could assess the error rate of the parametric and non-parametric methods. In addition, we repeated the simulations for three alpha levels (decision criterion of the system). The latter variable must be included because all of the four measures of accuracy we chose depend on the decision criterion used (Swets & Pickett, 1982). Therefore we need to monitor the error rate as a function of alpha. Finally, two simulations for all the above conditions are needed with one evaluating the right-handed test, and the other evaluating the left-handed test. The reason for this further splitting is that, as we have shown above in the case of skewed distributions, the parametric method generates two different types of error at the two sides of the distribution and we do not want to confuse them considering the outcomes of a two-sided test.

A total of 486 ($9 \times 9 \times 3 \times 2$) simulations were performed, each one evaluating 100,000 simulation entries. The simulations were performed by a computer program written in Delphi Pascal (Borland Corporation). All together they required approximately four hours computation time on a Dell personal computer equipped with a 1.8 GHz Pentium 4 processor and 512 Mb of RAM. Normative samples, the x_d vector described above, were emulated by means of a gaussian random number generator function embedded in Delphi Pascal. The function (called randG) generates random samples gaussian-distributed with a specified mean and standard deviation. For all simulations we used mean = 10 and variance = 1. In this way all random samples were non-negative. This was required by the skewness manipulation we chose (performed by means of a power transformation as seen below). Each distribution actually employed in the simulation was computed as the (sorted sample-by-sample) average of 10,000 gaussian distributions generated with the randG function. This ensured that correspondent distributions were very similar across different conditions of the simulation.

Alpha Level Manipulation

The alpha level is the decision criterion employed in the normative database. It quantifies the amount of evidence requested by the system before a positive outcome is issued. Three alpha levels were considered: 0.05, 0.025, and 0.0125. Since all tests were one-tailed, these three levels correspond to the two-tailed test alpha levels 0.01, 0.05, 0.025. Published databases considered in our review (e.g., Bosch-Bayard et al., 2001; John et al., 1987; Thatcher, 1999; Veldhuizen et al., 1993) use the fixed alpha level 0.05. In our simulations this corresponds to alpha = 0.025. In addition to this alpha level we considered a more stringent criterion (alpha = 0.0125), and a more lenient criterion (alpha = 0.05). The reason is that the measures of accuracy we used are independent of the prior probabilities of positive or negative events, but are not independent of the decision criterion (Swets & Pickett, 1982). Since we expect different error rates solely because the decision criterion is changed, we might want to monitor the behavior of our system as a function of the decision criterion.

Sample Size Manipulation

Nine sample sizes were considered, ranging from 80 to 720 with an increment of 80 (80, 160, 240, 320, 400, 480, 560, 640, 720). The choice for the increment was contingent. It can be shown that the accuracy of the non-parametric method for the minimum alpha level we considered (alpha = 0.0125) increases discretely in steps of 80 (sample size). The reason is intuitive. We show that the RV sample proportion (Φ) can take on only discrete values ranging between 0 and 1 increasing by a factor of 1/N. Consider the alpha level alpha = 0.0125. With N = 80, the possible values that the RV Φ can take, sorting them in ascending order, are 0, 0.0125, . . . 1. With N = 160, they will be 0, 0.00625, 0.0125, . . . 1. As soon as N reaches 160, the random variable Φ gains resolution, having the ability to take on three possible values less than the alpha level (p < alpha).

Gaussianity Manipulation

Gaussianity was manipulated transforming the normal averaged distribution with a power function. For each level of gaussianity considered each sample of the normative distribution was raised to a fixed power. This resulted in a skewed distribution respecting the order of the original samples. Nine levels of gaussianity were considered, corresponding to nine different powers ranging from 1 to 3 with an increment of 0.25 (1, 1.25, 1.5, 1.75, 2, 2.25, 2.5, 2.75, 3). The first distribution always remained unchanged after transformation (power of 1) and constituted a true empirical random gaussian distribution. In this case the performance of the parametric method was expected to be excellent. Table 3 reports the mean and standard deviations of the skewness and kurtosis of the empirical distributions actually used in the left-handed test and right-handed test simulations. Mean and standard deviations were computed across the different sample sizes used in the simulations for each level of the variable manipulating the gaussianity of the distribution. From Table 3 we can see that because of the averaging procedure, the gaussian random distributions all had very similar skewness and kurtosis for all the levels of sample size (small standard deviation), yielding almost identical distributions to be used in the left-handed test and right-handed test simulations. Table 3 also shows how skewness deteriorates with higher powers.

RESULTS

To capture the essence of our results we need to consider again Figure 2b. Let us anticipate the results for the parametric method. For a right-handed test, since the distribution has positive skewness, we expect three possible outcomes: E+|D+ (red area on the right of the distribution), E−|D+ (green area on the right of the distribution), and E−|D−

TABLE 3

Distribution	Mean Sk	Sd Sk	Mean Kt	Sd Kt
Pw of 1.00	0.000	0.002	2.869	0.085
Pw of 1.25	0.070	0.004	2.870	0.082
Pw of 1.50	0.140	0.006	2.884	0.084
Pw of 1.75	0.209	0.009	2.916	0.091
Pw of 2.00	0.279	0.010	2.962	0.093
Pw of 2.25	0.347	0.015	3.022	0.103
Pw of 2.50	0.417	0.017	3.100	0.113
Pw of 2.75	0.486	0.021	3.192	0.124
Pw of 3.00	0.556	0.024	3.299	0.137

Right-handed test

Distribution	Mean Sk	Sd Sk	Mean Kt	Sd Kt
Pw of 1.00	0.000	0.001	2.869	0.085
Pw of 1.25	0.070	0.004	2.870	0.083
Pw of 1.50	0.140	0.006	2.886	0.086
Pw of 1.75	0.210	0.008	2.916	0.089
Pw of 2.00	0.279	0.012	2.962	0.095
Pw of 2.25	0.348	0.015	3.026	0.102
Pw of 2.50	0.418	0.017	3.104	0.111
Pw of 2.75	0.486	0.021	3.193	0.125
Pw of 3.00	0.555	0.025	3.298	0.141

Left-handed test

(all the area left). The only discordant outcome (error) is the $E-|D+$ pairing. These are false positives. The error is due to the fact that although the area on the left of the observation is bigger than alpha ($E-$), the z-score computed with [1.0] is bigger than 1.96, leading to a p-value less than alpha ($D+$). Since this error happens on the right side we wish to compare it to the TP proportion. In other words (referring to Figure 2b), we wish to compare the green area (error) with the red area on its right. We will show that the specificity measure (SP) does not give us this information, but the true acceptance measure (TA) does. Remember that SP has been defined as TN/(FP+TN). Remember also that TN = $p(E-|D-)$ and FP = $p(E-|D+)$. In our simulations most entries are negative events. In fact the simulation entries were always random samples of the normative sample distribution. Hence (1-alpha)% of them is by definition a negative event and will fall in the $E-|D-$ (TN) category. The remaining will include $E+|D+$ and $E-|D+$ outcomes. Even if the FP proportion is large as compared to the TP proportion (the green area is big as compared to the red area) the specificity will be excellent, since it does not compare FP with TP, but FP with TN. On the other hand TA, defined as p(E+|D+), has as complement p(E−|D+). Its value is the right estimation of errors for this simulation (i.e., it compares the FP proportion to the TP proportion). This is the information we need. It is telling us among the events with positive diagnosis (green area + red area), how many, in proportion, were in reality positive (TP: red area) as compared to negative (FP: green area).

Consider next the left-handed test. Refer again to Figure 2b. Here we expect three different possible outcomes: E+|D+ (red area on the left of the distribution), E+|D− (green area on the left of the distribution), and E−|D− (all the area left). The only discordant outcome (error) is the E+|D− pairing (false negative), which is different from the type of error found on the right side. Here the error arises because although the area on the left of the observation is less than alpha (E+), the z-score computed with equation [1.0] is bigger than −1.96 (non-significant), leading to a p-value less than alpha (D−). We obtain some false negatives. Again, we wish to compare them to the TP proportion, and not to the TN proportion. In this case the sensitivity measure (SN) will give us this information. Remember that SN has been defined as TP/(TP+FN). Remember also that FN = p(E+|D−) and TP = p(E+|D+). For a left-handed text, (1-alpha)% of the outcomes will fall in the E−|D− category (notice that on this side of the distribution errors [FN] come at the expense of the TP proportion and the TN proportion is exactly [1-alpha]%). The remaining 5% will include E+|D+ and E+|D− outcomes. SN compares indeed TP to FN. This result is telling us that among the positive diagnosis how many, in proportion, were in reality positive events (TP) as compared with negative events (FN).

Errors with the non-parametric method follow a different pattern. For this method the appropriate measure of accuracy turns out to be the true acceptance (TA) for tests on both sides of the distribution. This means that for both the right-handed and left-handed test, the non-parametric method results in only three outcome pairings: the two concordant pairs E+|D+, E−|D−, and the discordant pair E−|D+. In other words, the non-parametric method tends to issue positive diagnosis when it is not the case.

In summary, considering that real normative distributions can be both left and right skewed, with the parametric method we expect both FP and FN errors depending on the side of the test and on the side of the skewness. With the non-parametric method we expect FP only, regardless the side of the test and the side of the skewness. We now show quantitative results of these errors. As expected, the accuracy of the parametric method was found to be the same (with little random error) at different sample sizes (N > 100) for all levels of non-gaussianity and alpha. Thus it will be shown as a function of non-gaussianity and alpha levels only. The accuracy of the non-parametric method was found to be the same (with little random error) at different non-gaussianity levels for all levels of sample size and alpha. Thus it will be shown as a function of sample size and alpha levels only. In every simulation performed, two out of the four measures of accuracy employed in this study always displayed a value of 1.0 (perfect accuracy) for all levels of the manipulated variable (i.e., they do not constitute a valuable test). The reason why this is the case has just been discussed. For example, for a right-handed test we do not expect false negatives for either method regardless the gaussianity, sample size, and alpha. Of the remaining two measures only the critical measure is reported. We have just seen that this is either the SN or the TA for the parametric method, and the TA for the non-parametric method. The critical measure always displayed values of accuracy less then or equal to 1.0 and changed monotonically across the levels of the manipulated variables.

Right-Handed Test

Results for the right-handed test are reported in Figure 3. Figure 3a refers to the parametric method (PM), while Figure 3b refers to the non-parametric method (nPM). The blue lines indicate the 0.95 level of a measure of accuracy. This level of accuracy can be considered excellent for any diagnostic system. The red lines indicate the 0.85 level of a measure of accuracy. This level of accuracy can be considered the minimum required for a normative database. Figure 3a reports the PM true acceptance (TA) proportion as a function of gaussianity of the normative reference sample (x-axis) for the three alpha levels employed. As explained in the above discussion, this is the critical test for the parametric method for a right-handed test when the reference distribution is right skewed. The TA is excellent in the case of normality of the reference distribution (power of 1) and deteriorates rapidly as the power increases; for power > 1.5 the TA proportion for the usual alpha level (0.025) is unacceptable (< 0.85). The critical test of the nPM method under identical conditions is shown in Figure 3b. This graph plots the TA proportion as a function of the sample size. As expected, the perfor-

FIGURE 3. Results of the simulations for the RIGHT-HANDED test. Reported on the vertical axis are the true acceptance (a) for the parametric method, and the true acceptance (b) for the non-parametric method. For the parametric method results are shown as a function of non-gaussianity (horizontal axis) of the normative reference distribution and alpha level (a). For the non-parametric method results are shown as a function of sample size (horizontal axis) and alpha level (b). The green line indicates where the measure of accuracy is equal to 0.95 (very good level of accuracy). The red line indicates where the measure of accuracy is equal to 0.85 (acceptable level of accuracy).

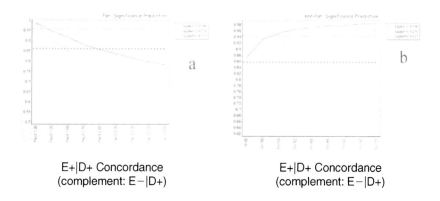

| E+\|D+ Concordance | E+\|D+ Concordance |
| (complement: E−\|D+) | (complement: E−\|D+) |

mance of the nPM increases monotonically with N. For the usual alpha level (0.025), the performance is acceptable (TA > 0.85) for N = 160, and excellent (TA > 0.95) for N = 400 or more.

Left-Handed Test

Results for the right-handed test are reported in Figure 4. Figure 4a refers to the parametric method (PM), while Figure 4b refers to the non-parametric method (nPM). The blue lines indicate the 0.95 level of a measure of accuracy. This level of accuracy would be considered excellent for any diagnostic system. The red lines indicate the 0.85 level of a measure of accuracy. This level of accuracy can be considered the minimum required for a normative database. Figure 4a reports the PM Sensitivity (SN) proportion as a function of gaussianity of the normative reference sample (x-axis) for the three alpha levels employed. As explained in the above discussion this is the critical test for the parametric method for a left-handed test, when the reference distribution is right skewed. The SN is excellent in the case of normality of the reference distribution (power of 1) but deteriorates rapidly as the power increases.

FIGURE 4. Results of the simulations for the LEFT-HANDED test. Reported on the vertical axis are the sensitivity (a) for the parametric method, and the proportion of true acceptance (b) for the non-parametric method. For the parametric method results are shown as a function of non-gaussianity (horizontal axis) of the normative reference distribution and alpha level (a). For the non-parametric method results are shown as a function of sample size (horizontal axis) and alpha level (b). The green line indicates where the measure of accuracy is equal to 0.95 (very good level of accuracy). The red line indicates where the measure of accuracy is equal to 0.85 (acceptable level of accuracy).

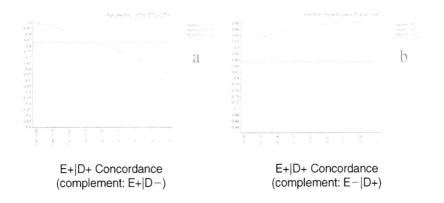

E+|D+ Concordance
(complement: E+|D−)

E+|D+ Concordance
(complement: E−|D+)

The decline is faster for the left-handed test than for the right-handed test (compare with Figure 3a). This phenomenon can easily be captured inspecting the two tails of the distribution in Figure 2b and considering the definition of SN and TA. On the left side errors (green area) grow at the expense of the true positive proportion (red area), while on the right side errors (green area) grow at the expense of the true negative proportion (all the area remaining on the left of the green area). The true positive proportion (red area) remains unchanged. For power > 1.25 the SN proportion for the usual alpha level (0.025) is already unacceptable (< 0.85). The critical test of the nPM method under identical conditions is shown in Figure 4b. This graph plots the TA proportion as a function of the sample size. As for the right-handed test, the performance of the nPM increases monotonically with N. For the usual alpha level (0.025), the performance is acceptable (TA > 0.85) for N = 160, and excellent (TA > 0.95) for N = 480 or above. Allowing few random errors, these results for the nPM are comparable to those obtained for the right-handed test. In fact the nPM performs equally at both sides of the distribution, no matter what the skewness is.

CONCLUSIONS

A total of 486 simulations were performed in order to compare two methods for the comparisons to EEG norms. The parametric method is based on z-scores and has been employed so far. The non-parametric method is based on sample proportions or, equivalently, percentiles and has been proposed in this paper to overcome some problems related with the use of the parametric method. Each simulation estimated the error rate in the diagnostic predictability of the two methods for both left-handed and right-handed tests. Variables manipulated included the decision criterion of the normative database (alpha level), sample size, and non-gaussianity of the normative reference sample. For each combination of the side of the test and the method employed, the critical test was individuated. This was one of the four accuracy measures considered in this study [sensitivity (SN), specificity (SP), true acceptance (TA), and true rejection (TR)]. The performance on the critical tests provided a framework for comparing the two methods. The performance of the parametric method (PM) was found to be unrelated to the sample size, given that N is not too small. With N < 80 the performance of the method starts deteriorating, therefore we conclude that this independence is true for approximately N > 100. The performance of the parametric method was found related to the non-gaussianity of the normative sample distribution. Empirical distributions for which the parametric performance can be considered acceptable have to be very close to a true theoretical gaussian distribution.

The performance of the non-parametric method was unaffected by the non-gaussianity of the normative reference distribution but was affected by the sample size. Acceptable (> 0.85) accuracy (enough resolution) can be attained with N = 160. Excellent accuracy (> 0.95) can be attained with no less than around 440 subjects. This result contradicts the common notion that non-parametric statistics "should be used with a small sample size." For both methods and for both the right-handed and left-handed tests, the critical tests result in less accuracy the smaller the decision criterion (alpha level). This important result contradicts the intuitive notion that reducing the alpha level would lead to a smaller rate of false positives. This is definitely not the case. Indeed alpha affects positively all measures of accuracy proportionally to its value; the bigger the alpha level, the better the accuracy. This result is explained with a specific example. The reasoning extends readily to all possible situations. Consider the left-handed test for the parametric test. The critical test for this situation is the sensitivity (SN). Remember the SN is defined as TP/(TP+FN) and that under these circumstances the database is going to issue only TP, FN and TN outcomes. SN increases proportionally as TP increases and as FN decreases. Refer to Figure 2b and look at the left tail of the distribution. This figure refers to a one-handed alpha level equal to 0.025. Imagine we halve the alpha level. Both the green area under the curve (FN) and the red area under the curve (TP) will decrease (they will be displaced on the left and here the height of the curve is smaller). However the red area will decrease more than the green area, the reason being that the curve is shorter at the left extremity. As a result, the ratio TP(TP+FN) will be smaller (i.e., sensitivity will be smaller). Doubling the alpha level, on the contrary, will result in a sensitivity increase.

Implications of Our Simulations for Database Development

We have been shown by means of simulations that the performance of the parametric test is impaired as a function of skewness. Nongaussianity due to high or low kurtosis is known to affect the test even more (Pollock, Schneider, & Lyness, 1990). These results are not a surprise. The problem is to assess how good the approximation to gaussianity for QEEG and ET the data is, and to evaluate the advantages acquired by using an alternative method. Regarding the approximation to gaussianity the literature is scattered and inconsistent. Only a few studies have been done investigating specifically the gaussiantity approximation for QEEG data and none, to our knowledge, have investigated the gaussianity approximation for electromagnetic tomographic (LORETA) data. Nonetheless the same transformations applied for QEEG measures have recently been applied to this kind of data to generate a normative database (Bosch-Bayard et al., 2001).

Electroencephalographic data in the frequency domain is markedly non-gaussian. Each measure is distributed in a particular way and the theoretical studies on their distribution are not exhaustive. For example, the power spectrum (absolute power) is distributed approximately as a chi-square (Beauchamp, 1973; Brillinger, 1975). The degrees of freedom (df) are a function of the EEG recording length (number of epochs), the FFT frequency resolution, wideness of the frequency bands considered, the time-domain tapering employed, and other technical factors. One should take into consideration all these factors in estimating the df associated with a power spectrum chi-square distribution. At the time when the databases were first developed (1970s) a simpler approach was employed. For each measure a suitable data transformation (based on log transformations) was used to approximate gaussianity. The idea was to allow a general method for the assessment of the deviance from the norms and also to allow parametric statistics to be employed in research comparing different groups. A few specific studies provided evidence of the appropriateness of these transformations (Gasser et al., 1982; Oken & Chiappa, 1988; Pollock et al., 1990). Other evidence has been provided in papers describing the construction of normative databases, but they are not as stringent from a statistical point of view (e.g., John et al., 1988).

A review of the literature and a close analysis of a large normative database convinced us that the gaussian approximation is not good enough to allow the use of parametric statistics. All specific studies found that the log-based transformations approximate gaussianity fairly well, but all of them found exceptions. Gasser et al. (1982) found exceptions in delta, theta, beta 1 and beta 2 for the absolute power measures. Oaken and Chiappa (1988) found that approximately one-eighth of the descriptors for absolute power remain non-gaussian after transformation. Relative power behaved a little better. Pollock et al. (1990) found the transformation of amplitude (square root of absolute power) to be excellent in all frequency bands but in theta. While John and his colleagues (1987, 1988) insist on data transformation, Thatcher (1998) found that for all measures, with the exception of phase, the untransformed data approximated gaussianity better than the transformed data, contradicting all previous results. It is worth noting that the sample size used in the John and Thatcher studies was similar, so the unreliability of results cannot be explained by means of "deus ex machina" such as the central limit theorem. Furthermore, all of these studies used different montages, electrode reference, age range of subjects and even different measures. Finally, if in the case of QEEG a few proportions of departure from gaussianity can be ignored, for electromagnetic tomography (LORETA) data it cannot be done capriciously.

Before compiling a parametric database one has to check that the distribution for all descriptors is approximately gaussian. In the case of ET data this involves tens of thousands of checks. With such a large number and all the variability of EEG data, many of them will not pass the tests. The question is how should one deal with them? Should the non-gaussian descriptors be excluded from the database? Even ignoring this problem, we will be left with a normative database in which accuracy is different for each descriptor. In fact, we have shown that the accuracy is a function of skewness and each approximation to gaussianity will lead to different skewness levels. Furthermore, the outcome of the normative database will be different on the two sides of the distribution. These are not desirable characteristics for a normative database. One may overcome all of these problems by using a non-parametric approach, given that the sample size is large enough. It is fortunate that normative databases of clinical usefulness are constructed on the basis of large samples. Actually the sample sizes commonly employed are so large (500-600) that they would lead to more than 96% accuracy if the non-parametric method described in this article was employed. Furthermore, the validity of results would be the same for the right-handed and the left-handed test, for all electrodes, frequency bands and for whatever measure is employed regardless of its distribution. In fact the sample size is the only true constant across descriptors. We have shown in this article that the accuracy of the non-parametric method, given a fixed alpha level, depends solely on sample size. This is the distinct advantage of the non-parametric method. The extension of the non-parametric method to ET data and to new electroencephalographic measures is straightforward. We also contend that developmental equations and other kinds of between-subject differences can be taken into account while compiling a non-parametric normative database. For instance, polynomial regression equations based on age can be computed. Each descriptor value can be normalized over its predicted value to remove any unwanted trend in the data. In the 1970s it was not easy to perform a non-parametric test. Computers were slow and the computations required could took hours. Today they would take minutes. Another possible reason why non-parametric methods have not been employed is that they require more intense computer programming. However one does not have to check data gaussianity, nor struggle to find appropriate data transformation, nor be concerned about the distribution of new measures any longer. By using a non-parametric method one would actually maximize resources and the prediction of clinical versus non-clinical membership would be improved.

REFERENCES

Ahn, H., Prichep, L. S., John, E. R., Baird, H., Trepetin, & Kaye, H. (1980). Developmental equations reflect brain dysfunctions. *Science, 210*, 1259-1262.

Beauchamp, K. G. (1973). *Signal processing using analog and digital techniques.* London: George Allen & Unwin.

Brillinger, D. R. (1975). *Time series: Data analysis and theory.* New York: Holt, Rinehart, and Winston.

Bosch-Bayard, J., Valdés-Sosa, P., Virues-Alba, T., Aubert-Vázquez, E., John, E. R., Harmony, T. et al. (2001). 3D statistical parametric mapping of EEG source spectra by means of variable resolution electromagnetic tomography (VARETA). *Clinical Electroencephalography, 32*, 47-61.

Duffy, F. H., Bartels, P. H., & Burchfiel, J. L. (1981). Significance probability mapping: An aid in the topographic analysis of brain electrical activity. *Electroencephalography and Clinical Neurophysiology, 51*, 455-462.

Fuchs, M., Wagner, M., Köhler, T., & Wischmann, H. A. (1999). Linear and nonlinear current density reconstructions. *Journal of Clinical Neurophysiology, 16*, 267-295.

Gasser, T., Bächer, P., & Möcks, J. (1982). Transformation towards the normal distribution of broad band spectral parameters of the EEG. *Electroencephalography and Clinical Neurophysiology, 53*, 119-124.

Gasser, T., Verleger, R., Bächer, P., & Sroka, L. (1988). Development of the EEG of school-age children and adolescents. I. Analysis of band power. *Electroencephalography and Clinical Neurophysiology, 69*, 91-99.

Guggenmoos-Holzman, I., & van Houwelingen, H. C. (2000). The (in)validity of sensitivity and specificity. *Statistics in Medicine, 19*, 1783-1792.

Hernández, J. L., Valdés, P., Biscay, R., Virues, T., Szava, S., Bosch, J. et al. (1994). A global scale factor in brain. *International Journal of Neorosciences, 76*, 267-278.

Holmes, A. P., Blair, R. C., Watson, J. D. G., & Ford, I. (1996). Nonparametric analysis of statistic images from functional mapping experiments. *Journal of Cerebral Blood-Flow Metabolism, 16*, 7-22.

Hughes, J. R., & John, E. R. (1999). Conventional and quantitative electroencephalography in psychiatry. *Journal of Neuropsychiatry and Clinical Neuroscience, 11*, 190-208.

John, E. R., Karmel, B., Corning, W., Easton, P., Brown, D., Ahn, H. et al. (1977). Neurometrics: Numerical taxonomy identifies different profiles of brain functions within groups of behaviorally similar people. *Science, 196*, 1393-1410.

John, E. R., Ahn, H., Prichep, L. S., Trepetin, M., Brown, D., & Kaye, H. (1980a). Developmental equations for the electroencephalogram. *Science, 210*, 1255-1258.

John, E. R., Karmel, B. Z., Corning, W. C., Easton, P., Brown, D., Ahn, H. et al. (1980b). Neurometrics. *Science, 196*, 1393-1409.

John, E. R., Prichep, L. S., & Easton, P. (1987). Normative data banks and neurometrics: Basic concepts, method and results of norm constructions. In A. S. Gevins & A. Remond (Eds.), *Method of analysis of brain electrical and magnetic signals: Vol. 1. EEG handbook* (revised series, pp. 449-495). New York: Elsevier Science Publishers B. V. (Biomedical Division).

John, E. R., Prichep, L. S., Fridman, J., & Easton, P. (1988). Neurometrics: Computer assisted differential diagnosis of brain dysfunctions. *Science, 239*, 162-169.

Lipschutz, S., & Lipson, M .L. (2000). *Probability. Schaum's outline series* (2nd ed.). New York: McGraw-Hill.

Lunneborg, C. E. (1999). *Data analysis by resampling: Concepts and applications.* Pacific Grove, CA: Duxbury Press.

Lynn, P. A., & Fuerst, W. (1989). *Introductory digital signal processing with computer applications.* New York: John Wiley & Sons.

Matthis, P., Scheffner, D., Benninger, C., Lipinsky, C., & Stolzis, L. (1980). Changes in the background activity of the electroencephalogram according to age. *Electroencephalography and Clinical Neurophysiology, 49,* 626-635.

Nuwer, M. R. (1988). Quantitative EEG: II. Frequency analysis and topographic mapping in clinical settings. *Journal of Clinical Neurophysiology, 5,* 45-85.

Oken, B. S., & Chiappa, K. H. (1988). Short-term variability in EEG frequency analysis. *Electroencephalography and Clinical Neurophysiology, 69,* 191-198.

Pascual-Marqui, R. D. (1995). Reply to comments by Hämäläinen, Ilmoniemi and Nunez. In W. Skrandies (Ed.), *Source localization: Continuing discussion of the inverse problem. ISBET Newsletter, 6,* 16-28.

Pascual-Marqui, R. D. (1999). Review of methods for solving the EEG inverse problem. *International Journal of Bioelectromagnetism, 1,* 75-86.

Pascual-Marqui, R. D., Michel, C. M., & Lehmann, D. (1994). Low resolution electromagnetic tomography: A new method for localizing electrical activity in the brain. *International Journal of Psychophysiology, 18,* 49-65.

Pollock, V. E., Schneider, L. S., & Lyness, S. A. (1990). EEG amplitude in healthy, late-middle-aged and elderly adults: Normality of the distributions and correlation with age. *Electroencephalography and Clinical Neurophysiology, 75,* 276-288.

Swets, J. A. (1988). Measuring the accuracy of diagnostic systems. *Science, 240,* 1285-1293.

Swets, J. A., & Pickett, R. M. (1982). *Evaluation of diagnostic systems: Methods from signal detection theory.* New York: Academic Press.

Szava, S., Valdes, P., Biscay, R., Galan, L., Bosch, J., Clark, I. et al. (1994). High resolution quantitative EEG analysis. *Brain Topography, 6,* 211, 219.

Talairach, J, & Tournoux, P. (1988). *Co-planar stereotaxic atlas of the human brain.* New York: Thieme Medical Publishers.

Thatcher, R. W. (1998). EEG normative databases and EEG biofeedback. *Journal of Neurotherapy, 2* (4), 8-39.

Thatcher, R. W. (1999). EEG database-guided neurotherapy. In J. R. Evans & A. Abarbanel (Eds.), *Quantitative EEG and neurofeedback* (pp. 29-64). San Diego, CA: Academic Press.

van Beijsterveldt, C. E. M., Molenaar, P. C. M., de Gaus, E. J. C., & Boosma, D. I. (1996). Heritability of human brain functioning as assessed by electroencephalography. *American Journal of Human Genetics, 58,* 562-573.

Veldhuizen, R. J., Jonkman, E. J., & Poortvliet, D. C. J. (1993). Sex differences in age regression parameters of healthy adults-normative data and practical implications. *Electroencephalography and Clinical Neurophysiology, 86,* 377-384.

Use of Databases in QEEG Evaluation

Jack Johnstone, PhD
Jay Gunkelman, QEEG-D

SUMMARY. *Background.* Quantitative electroencephalography (qEEG) analysis incorporating the use of normative or reference database comparison has developed from being primarily a research tool into an increasingly widely used method for clinical neurophysiological evaluation.

Method. A survey of several of the most widely used qEEG databases as well as issues surrounding the construction and use of these databases is presented, comparing and contrasting the various features of these databases, followed by a discussion of critical issues in this developing technology.

Results. This review considers the concept of normalcy, norming of qEEG features, and validation of clinical findings. Technical issues such as methods for recording and analysis, filter use, broad bands versus single Hz finer frequency resolution, the number of variables relative to the number of cases, and the problem of multiple statistical testing are addressed. The importance of the recording electrode and montage reformatting for normative EEG data is emphasized. The use of multiple references is suggested.

Discussion. A brief review of the characteristics of several major da-

Jack Johnstone is President and CEO, and Jay Gunkelman is Executive Vice President, Q-Metrx, Inc., Burbank, CA.

Address correspondence to: Jack Johnstone, President, Q-Metrx, Inc., 2701 West Alameda Avenue, Suite 304, Burbank, CA 91505.

tabases is presented. Each has advantages and disadvantages, and newer databases will exploit new technological developments and increasing sophistication in statistical analysis of EEG data. Implementing new measures such as variability over time and extraction of features such as event-related desynchronization (see Pfurtscheller, Maresch, & Schuy, 1985) and gamma synchrony (Rennie, Wright, & Robinson, 2000) are likely to have important clinical impact. Caution is urged in the use of automated classification by discriminant analysis. *[Article copies available for a fee from The Haworth Document Delivery Service: 1-800-HAWORTH. E-mail address: <docdelivery@haworthpress.com> Website: <http://www. HaworthPress.com> © 2003 by The Haworth Press, Inc. All rights reserved.]*

KEYWORDS. qEEG, databases, normalcy, montage reformatting, Laplacian, discriminant analysis

INTRODUCTION

Quantitative electroencephalography (qEEG) analysis refers to signal processing and extraction of features from the EEG signal. In typical practice, multichannel EEG is digitized, edited or adjusted to remove extra cerebral artifact, and subjected to spectral analysis using the fast Fourier transform (FFT). Extraction of features such as amount of power at each electrode for each frequency band or coherence among channels as a function of frequency is carried out for an individual and then compared to a "normal" group or another clinically defined group.

The use of a database has become an integral part of qEEG reporting, which usually also includes topographic color-graduated representation of EEG features (Duffy, Burchfiel, & Lombroso, 1979). Another important component of the qEEG study is visual inspection of the raw waveforms by a clinically experienced electroencephalographer (Duffy, Hughes, Miranda, Bernad, & Cook, 1994). Visual inspection of the EEG data is required to identify the possible presence of significant transient events as well as to evaluate transitions evolving over time, and assess the influence of extracerebral artifacts on the record.

There are many issues to be considered in construction and use of a comparison database in the clinical assessment of individuals. This review will be concerned with problems such as the definition of normalcy, how individuals are recruited and screened for inclusion in the database, types of EEG features that are normed, and the use of statistical analysis of EEG data. It is important to consider the specific reason for use of database comparisons. Frequency tuning in neurofeedback applications may require analysis and display of single Hz information, while other applications (medical, legal, pharmacologic) may have different requirements. A comprehensive database should allow for a number of applications. Several databases currently in use will be examined with respect to these issues.

NORMALCY

The definition of a database as a representation of the range of "normal" within a population raises the issue of what is meant by normal. A database could be comprised of many individuals in a population who are not rigorously screened for neuropsychiatric disorders, space occupying lesions, or aberrant neurophysiological functioning. If the population is very large, a simple statistical definition could be applied with those individuals falling close to the mean of a particular variable considered as normal and those with deviant scores considered abnormal. That is, the normal group falls within the bell shape of the normal curve and the abnormal group at the tails. Of course the problem here is that an individual may fall close to the mean for one variable but not other variables. A "pure" normal would be close to the mean for *all* variables. It is important to keep in mind that deviations from a database represent differences from average, not from optimal.

This is different from a clinically normal database where individuals are carefully screened for relevant abnormalities using other clinical tools such as psychometric assessment or MRI. In common clinical practice clinical and statistical deviation are often combined with limited screening (e.g., questionnaires) and statistical significance assessed conservatively (e.g., greater than three standard deviations from the mean). Further, there are technical concerns about calling a database representative of the normal population. To truly represent a particular population, stratified sampling must be employed. The database should represent the mix of ages, gender, ethnicity, socioeconomic status and other demographic factors present in the overall population. Most databases in current use in qEEG do not meet criteria for this level of norming, and are more appropriately considered reference rather than normative databases. Using a rigorously screened population, deviations represent the difference from well functioning as compared to average.

The method of recruitment of putatively normal individuals also should be considered. Often laboratory or office personnel are designated as normal because of good work skills and are used to populate the database. We have seen repeated occurrences of abnormal test results from office personnel who with sufficient questioning admit to occasional migraine headache or use of over the counter medications, etc. This points to the danger of poor screening procedures resulting in admitting individuals into a normal group who have significant clinical problems. When advertisements are used and paid volunteers are recruited, care must be exercised not to entice individuals to participate and falsify information because of the financial reward. We have advertised for boys to participate in a brain wave study and had parents bring in children that they suspected as having neurological or psychiatric problems for the hidden purpose of obtaining a free evaluation.

With respect to the extent of screening required to construct a proper database of normal individuals, certain practical constraints are relevant. It would be desirable to have full MRI, PET, fMRI, complete neuropsychological evaluation, genetic analysis, blood and urine testing, etc., but this may be prohibitively time consuming and costly. We argue that some form of screening is useful beyond simple self-report measures, which are well known to be unreliable. In addition to questionnaire information, objective assessment of general health, social and intellectual functioning is critical.

Special concerns apply to pediatric databases where dramatic developmental changes occur over relatively short time intervals. It is inappropriate to compare a four-year-old patient to norms derived from six-year-olds. The same two-year difference would be trivial in adults. It is possible to compute developmental equations over a relatively wide age range in childhood that reflects normal changes in development (Ahn et al., 1980). Departure from the normal trajectory of development of particular qEEG features could be considered a potentially clinically relevant finding. The size of the population required for computation of a stable set of developmental equations depends on the number of qEEG variables being studied. The larger the *cases to variables ratio*, the more stable and reliable the assessment. The number of subjects needed in a given database is larger as more measures are normed in order to account for use of multiple statistical tests.

NORMING EEG FEATURES

Evaluation of the pattern of deviations compared to a reference database is typically an integral part of qEEG evaluation. Most often a set of parametric univariate Z-scores is computed as a way of detecting and characterizing potential abnormalities. The use of parametric statistics assumes a normal (gaussian) distribution of the variable(s) in question. Data transformation (log, square root, etc.) may be useful in meeting assumptions of parametric statistics. In addition, further exploration of other statistical methods (e.g., nonparametric) may be useful for application to the special requirements of EEG data.

It is not strictly the number of deviations, rather the *pattern* of deviations that is most relevant. Most database analyses do not allow for quantitative multivariate assessment of such patterns, and the overall pattern of significance must be reviewed by an individual with relevant experience in EEG, and both clinical and statistical evaluation. John et al. (1983) describe the use of the Mahalanobis distance statistic to capture patterns of regional deviation, for example, deviations involving the entire the left lateral or anterior brain regions.

Spectral power is an often used measure in qEEG studies. The amount of power for each frequency or frequency band for a given electrode is computed and compared to the database mean value. The results are usually represented as Z-scores, which is the difference between the mean score of a population and the patient's individual score divided by the standard deviation of the population.

There is a clear trend in the field toward more recording electrodes. Many recording systems now offer 32 to 40 channels. Further, using faster sampling rates, wider band passes (e.g., increasing the frequency setting of the high frequency filter), and higher resolution analog to digital conversion (A/D) allows for a more complete evaluation of the EEG signal over a wider range of frequencies. It is expected that new databases will provide norms past the 40 Hz range. The number of Z-scores increases as the number of electrodes, frequency bands, and recording conditions increases. The use of a large number of variables without corresponding increases in the sample size of the normal population increases the likelihood of deviation occurring by chance, unrelated to true neurophysiological abnormality. The number of false positive findings can be limited by requiring replication of patterns of deviation on independent samples of individual patient data.

Most databases available for clinical use contain the mean values of particular EEG features and the standard deviation of the feature across the normal population (see John, Prichep, & Easton, 1987). Certain databases provide not only spectral power (or magnitude, the square root of power) but other derived measures such as relative power. Relative power represents the percentage of power in any bands compared with the total power in the patient's EEG (e.g., relative theta is the percentage of theta of the combined sum of delta, theta, alpha, and beta). Other derived measures that have been normed include hemispheric asymmetry for power: comparing homologous electrode sites over the two hemispheres, as well as anterior/posterior power gradients. It should be recognized that these measures are not statistically independent, and significant deviations on more than one feature may be representing the same neurophysiological process.

Derived EEG features also include correlation or similarity measures such as coherence or the cross-spectrum, sometimes referred to as the comodulation (Sterman & Kaiser, 2001). These measures index the similarity of activity between two recordings. When two electrodes are placed closely together on the scalp they pick up a large amount of common signal and recordings are highly correlated. Database comparisons are useful in showing when the signals are too correlated or not correlated enough as a function of the distance between the recording electrodes.

Phase measures the time delay between activities at two sites. The phase measures have also been normed. It is clear that phase is an important measure in understanding propagation of neuronal activity. Progressive phase delays are measurable as a volley travels from a source to a destination. In addition, 180 degree differences in phase denote polarity inversion and suggest the location of underlying generators. Using polarity inversion to model the source of brain macropotentials is useful in localizing activity and is commonly used in electroencephalography (Niedermeyer & Lopes da Silva, 1999). However, the meaning and utility of measures of average phase over time is not as clear.

Nearly all databases utilize features extracted in the frequency domain. Phase is a measure of timing derived from frequency domain analysis. It is also possible to norm measures directly in the time domain. The sequence and timing of neuronal activities following sensory stimulation can be measured very precisely and the timing and sequence of these events can be normed. Time domain analysis usually is carried out on the average response to the presentation of many sensory stimuli, the so-called averaged evoked potential (EP) or event-related potential (ERP; see Misulis & Fakhoury, 2001). Time domain techniques are very powerful in minimizing extra cerebral artifact not specifically linked to the presentation of the sensory stimuli. The ERP method is therefore a good candidate for recording under conditions of increased artifact, such as performance of complex psychomotor tasks.

The P300 is a well-characterized component of the ERP (for example, see Donchin, 1987). The usual procedure involves presentation of many standard stimuli, intermixed with occasional target stimuli. The stimuli are most often auditory tones or clicks but the procedure works generally independent of the sensory modality. The recognition of targets embedded in a series of standard stimuli is accompanied by a positive-wave recorded from the scalp at about 300 milliseconds following the stimulus, called the P300. The size and timing of the P300 component of the ERP is sensitive to the detectability of the stimulus, the speed of presentation, and a host of patient alerting, attentional and memory processes. We advocate the use of the P300 as a sort of treadmill test. The ability of a patient to detect and respond to increasingly difficult stimuli will be reflected in the timing (latency) and size (amplitude) of the P300. It is possible to determine at what point the P300 changes in character for a given individual responding to the increasing challenge of the P300 task. Norming this type of feature should provide a more robust measure of brain activity under stress because of the suppression of artifact by signal averaging. This procedure appears more amenable to routine clinical evaluation than presentation of complex tasks such as reading or math where frequency domain analysis is often so severely contaminated by muscle, eye motion, and other movement artifact that data are unable to be interpreted.

A problem with most of the currently available databases is the sole reliance on the linked ear reference. Often this reference is not only active but asymmetric. Problems using a single linked ear reference point for all analyses can be reduced by use of multiple references and by montage reformatting, as described below.

MONTAGE REFORMATTING

To record an EEG a multichannel recording amplifier is used. Each channel has a differential preamplifier, which has three electrical contacts: a ground contact, typically via a system or chassis ground which has a ground electrode contact on the patient; the two other contacts go directly into the differential preamplifier (Tyner & Knott, 1983). The preamplifier amplifies the voltage (E) difference between two electrodes placed in the two inputs, which are designated as grid one (G1) and grid two (G2) in electronic terms. This may be expressed as the following equation:

EEG equals grid 1 voltage minus grid 2 voltage

$$EEG = G1(E) - G2(E)$$

These two inputs give the EEG preamplifier the differential voltage, which fluctuates, or oscillates, over time creating the EEG waveform. This is simply showing the first grid's input electrode activity with respect to the grid two electrode activity. These combinations of inputs, summed to show the whole set of electrodes being monitored, is called the montage (French for mountings). A montage is selected to most clearly demonstrate the EEG pattern being monitored. One example is the controversial "14 and 6 positive spikes," which are *visualized* in ear reference montages more clearly than with sequential montages, though focal spike discharges are more easily *localized* with the sequential montages or with Laplacian/Hjorth techniques (Scherg, Ille, Bornfleth, & Berg, 2002).

Many will refer to the active electrode (grid 1) and the reference electrode (grid 2). Commonly used references include the ear references (linked ear, ipsilateral and contralateral ear), the Cz or vertex reference, and the sequential references (commonly termed bipolar). A more modern reference is based on Laplacian mathematics; it is variously called the Hjorth reference, local average, reference free, and virtual reference. Other computerized references include the common average or global average and the weighted average reference (Scherg et al., 2002).

Some montages need to have special electrodes applied, though these montages are not the subject of this paper. These include some obscure placements such as the tip of nose, the mastoid process, as well as the more obscure sternum-spinal reference (which cancels the EKG), or the more invasive references used in epilepsy research (e.g., the naso-pharyngeal or sphenoid leads) as well as direct cortical measurement (see Niedermeyer & Lopes da Silva, 1999).

Though it might seem comforting to be told which montage is the "right one" or the "best" montage, this is a more complex issue. The montages all have significant strengths and weaknesses, with the benefit being the ability to customize the montage to fit the finding that needs to be displayed. The weakness of this flexibility is in missing or inadvertently trivializing a phenomenon, or even creating a false image in the EEG if the reference selected is not a relatively neutral area electrically. An example is when strong temporal alpha contaminates the mastoid due to the lateral spread of the EEG through the skull. Thus, the ear references when contaminated create false alpha, displaced to areas without alpha by the differential amplification system, which is blind as to the source of an oscillation, whether grid 1 or the reference at grid 2, the EEG output is an oscillation (see Gunkelman, 2000).

The selection of the montage needs to be based on the EEG but using a *variety* of montages is a part of the minimum guidelines for EEG, a guideline to which insurance companies can audit you for compliance. It is a commonly adopted guideline developed by the American Society of Electroneurodiagnostic Technologists. Their guidelines may be found on their web site (www.aset.org). This document also specifies 20 to 30 minutes of total recording time to meet these guidelines.

This practice of switching perspectives avoids the reader being fooled by a false localization when a reference is contaminated with voltages as described above. The montage is like a perspective, it is used to present information from a particular point of view.

Each montage has strengths as well as weaknesses, including the problem of the neutrality of the reference. A single ear reference will avoid any problem associated with the other ear's contamination though it does not cancel the EKG as well as the linked ear reference, as well as creating an apparent asymmetry due to the systematically different inter-electrode distances between the two hemispheres.

The Cz reference will give good resolution for the temporal areas but not the central area. The Cz montage is also a poor choice where there is drowsiness, with the associated vertex sharp waves and spindles which are seen maximally along the midline anteriorly and at the vertex which will contaminate the vertex electrode.

The sequential placements, whether anterior-posterior or transverse, all have good localization of cortical events through phase reversal, but the raw wave morphologies are distorted by the phase cancellations as well.

The linked ear montage is subject to temporal lobe activity being seen on the reference, likely via volumetric conduction from the temporal activity and the influences of lateral diffusion of activity seen with the skull. The activity seen at T5 and T6 are most likely to be seen in the electrodes on the ears but activity at T3 and T4 may be influential as well.

The Laplacian technique or local average (or the Hjorth) is quite good at showing localized findings. The Laplacian montages are effective in elimination of the cardioballistic artifacts. The Hjorth derivation will also make the focal nature of the electrode artifacts seen easily. This is often not used for display due to the unforgiving nature of the display. There is a minor distortion at the edge electrodes, commonly a small percentage error, though not a real problem for clinical utility. More problematic is the poor display of generalized or regional EEG findings, with false localization to the perimeter or edge of the finding (Scherg et al., 2002).

The global average is also a Laplacian technique, with the average of all electrodes used as the reference. This technique also has distortions when displaying generalized changes, especially generalized paroxysmal activity. This global reference may be done with a spatial weighting factor, which tunes the filter spatially to be more or less sensitive to focal findings. This weighted average reference is very popular when using dense arrays in topographic mapping.

One of the major factors in selecting montages is that the database selected has to have the same montage for the norms and to have any relevance to the data. Comparisons must be carried out with the same montage. This does not preclude reviewing the raw EEG data with these various montages, as well as creating topographic maps of these various montages to display the EEG, though it is mandatory that the proper montage be compared to the database.

The proper selection of montages will allow the reader to get a good view of the EEG phenomenon and its distribution across the cortex. Understanding of the topographic distribution of brain function is required to understand what the neuropsychological impacts of the EEG changes might be.

VALIDATION

In order to yield valid representations of neurophysiological abnormality by statistical deviation, the influence of artifact must be taken into account. Artifact can be generated by a variety of extra cerebral sources commonly including muscle, cardio-ballistic propagation, eye motion, sweat (GSR), and movement (see Hammond & Gunkelman, 2001). Since these artifacts occur to some extent in virtually all EEG recordings it is useful to specifically record and characterize the extent of artifacts. Concurrent recording of EMG, eye movement, and EKG are commonly used in EEG evaluation. High correlation between scalp recorded data and data from artifact channels increases the likelihood that the EEG is contaminated by artifact. The effects of correlated artifactual data can be reduced by statistically removing the signal using partial correlation. Although this is not commonly done, there is no substitute for making every attempt to minimize artifact at the time of the recording. It should be emphasized that at this time there are no validated procedures for automatic rejection of EEG artifact.

Another important influence on the EEG involves the effects of psychoactive medication. Normative databases do not include individuals taking medication whereas many if not most patients are taking medication, and often multiple medications, and in fact may not even report the use of over the counter medication or street drugs. Effects of medications are known to substantially alter the EEG frequency content, often causing large increases in slow or fast activity. The only methods useful in limiting these effects are (a) have a referring physician withdraw the medications prior to the test, which is generally not practical; or (b) take known effects of medications into account in the interpretation. It is clear that it is desirable to also verify medication status with drug screening for individuals included in a normal database.

A related issue involves non-medication supplements, or agents such as used in hormone replacement therapy. Since these agents replace normally occurring hormones it may not be necessary to consider them in the same way as pharmaceuticals in general. However, many replacements are synthetic and may not cause the same effects as naturally occurring hormones. Many vitamins, particularly b-vitamins, and nutriceuticals also have direct effects on the EEG.

Another difficult issue is the influence of patient drowsiness. Decreases in patient arousal and increased drowsiness can be expected routinely in EEG recording. These effects may be very subtle, and in fact may be the essence of the patient presentation and complaint. The individual recording the EEG should be aware of the common effects of mild drowsiness, namely a decrease in posterior alpha activity and increased slow activity, usually over the frontal midline. Attempts should be made to monitor for the effects of drowsiness and alert the patient as necessary at the time of the recording. Sophisticated and cost-effective monitors of the effects of drowsiness and loss of conscious awareness are now available and may be used concurrently to assure that the patient is alert, or if not, quantify the level of patient awareness (see Sigl & Chamoun, 1994; Johnstone, 2002).

A number of methods for deletion of artifact are available but automated methods are not generally used in clinical practice at this time. Typically, segments of EEG containing significant artifact are simply deleted from analysis based on visual inspection by a trained technician or clinical specialist.

In addition to validating the quality of EEG data, another type of clinical validation involves assuring that appropriate deviations occur with cases of known pathology, such as amplitude suppression of focal slowing post-stroke or diffuse excessive slow activity in advanced dementia.

DATABASES IN PRACTICE

Several databases are commercially available for clinical use. Several widely used databases have been reviewed and compared by Lorensen and Dickson (2001). Following is a brief review of several currently available databases and a description of a new multifactorial, comprehensive database currently under construction.

Neurometrics

The first database developed for the purpose of general neurophysiological evaluation was constructed by John, Prichep and Easton (1987). The term "neurometrics" was first used by this group to describe an analogy to psychometric assessment, commonly used in clinical psychology (John et al., 1977). Neurometrics refers to the comparison of individual EEG features with a reference database and is used in much the same way as IQ testing. A standardized test is constructed using a large population of individuals and the relative standing of the test results for a given individual within that overall population is assessed. John et al. (1987) stressed the need for standardization of recruitment, recording, and analysis procedures.

The Neurometric database is based on a specific set of EEG features: absolute power, relative power, coherence, mean frequency within band, and symmetry (left-right and front-back) extracted from approximately two minutes of data selected for being minimally contaminated by artifact. Only recordings made with eyes closed at rest were analyzed and normed. The EEG frequency range analyzed extends from .5 to 25 Hz. Extracted features were transformed to assure a gaussian (normal) distribution. Two thousand and eighty-four (2,084) variables are computed for each member of the database. The correlation of EEG features with age was noted and best fit age regression equations were developed to account for age effects. Univariate and multivariate Z-scores were computed for the purpose of characterizing an individual's deviations from the mean of the population. This database includes measures from some 782 normal individuals. Of this total 356 cases were between the ages of 6 to 16 and 426 cases were between the ages 16 to 90. Over

4,000 clinical cases were used in the discriminant section of the software.

Individuals selected for inclusion in the Neurometric database were screened by questionnaire to exclude head injury, neurological or psychiatric disease, any history of psychological problems, alcohol or drug abuse, any use of psychotropic medication, and academic or social problems.

One important feature of the Neurometric database is the availability of normed features for specific sequential (bipolar) electrode pairs. This feature allows for at least some assessment of the effects of activity recorded with the linked ear reference.

We have had extensive experience with the Neurometric database and have found it to be useful in both characterizing abnormalities detected by visual inspection, as well as in identifying patterns of deviation which appear to be clinically significant but are not easily detected by inspection of the raw EEG signals. We appreciate that the Neurometric database has received a 510(k) clearance by the FDA (July, 1998, #K974748), indicating that construction of the database has been scrutinized for good manufacturing practices (GMPs). The 510(k) also signifies the legitimacy of marketing claims made concerning the database.

The most significant problem with the Neurometric database is exclusive reliance on banded EEG. Only information about delta, theta, alpha, and low frequency beta bands are available. Findings restricted to narrow frequencies are often seen when data are displayed in single Hz increments but are obscured with the use of the relatively wide bands as normed in the Neurometric database.

Thatcher Lifespan Normative EEG Database (LSNDB/NeuroGuide)

The database developed by Robert W. Thatcher has been described in detail (Thatcher, 1998). Subsequently, during 1999-2000 new analyses presented under the commercial name "NeuroGuide" were completed (see *www.appliedneuroscience.com*). The lifespan database was reconstructed starting with the same raw digital EEG values from the same normal subjects. This database now contains information from 625 individuals, covering the age range two months to 82.6 years. More advanced methods were used to compute the revised database, including more extensive cross-validation and tests of gaussian distributions for average reference, linked ears, Laplacian, eyes open and eyes closed. The NeuroGuide database has been tested and re-tested and the sensitivity of the statistical distributions has been calculated for each montage and condition.

Normalcy was determined by response to a neurological history questionnaire which was given to the child's parents and/or filled out by each subject. IQ and other age appropriate psychometric testing, academic achievement, as well as class room performance as determined by school grades and teacher reports also were used in determining normalcy.

Nine hundred and forty-three (943) variables were computed for each subject including measures of absolute and relative power, coherence, phase, asymmetry, and power ratios. Z-score transforms are available in single Hz bins. Sliding averages were used to compute age-appropriate norms. Results were inspected for gaussian distribution. Recording with task challenges was not performed (for further details see Thatcher, Walker, Biver, North, & Curtin, Sensitivity and cross-validation of a lifespan normative EEG database at: *http://www.appliedneuroscience. com/LSNDBWEB.htm*).

NeuroGuide was considered to not require FDA 510(k) clearance, based on both the non-medical nature of the intended use and the fact that databases are considered tables of numbers involving library functions. Overall, the construction and composition of this database are relatively well documented.

Sterman-Kaiser (SKIL) Database

The SKIL database currently includes 135 adults ranging from 18 to 55 years old (see Sterman & Kaiser, 2001, Appendix: Adult Database Description, available at: *http://www.skiltopo.com/manual.htm*). No normative information is currently available for children or young adults, although data is being collected to cover the younger ages. SKIL does not consider age as a factor in computing Z-score deviations. The reference population is comprised of students and laboratory personnel (50%), volunteers recruited from the community (25%), and U.S. Air Force personnel (25%). Screening was based on questionnaires regarding medical history, drug use, and recent life events.

The SKIL database incorporates recordings at rest (eyes closed and open) and during task challenges involving audio-visual information processing and visual-spatial tracking. A correction for the time of day of recording is available which is based on combined cross-sectional and longitudinal data rather than the preferred method of tracking within-subject changes over time.

The SKIL database covers a restricted range of frequencies, from 2 to 25 Hz. This method deletes significant slow and fast frequency data which may be of clinical importance. However, the database does have the advantage of providing norms for each single Hz increment over this frequency range. The SKIL database relies exclusively on the linked ear reference. The SKIL analysis has not received FDA 510(k) clearance and is labeled as not intended for medical use.

The SKIL database does not have a measure of EEG coherence but rather includes a similarity measure termed comodulation, which is quite like coherence but does not yield a measure of phase. Comodulation is essentially the correlation of the spectrum for two recording electrodes over time using a sliding one second data window moved in 250 millisecond increments. Although this effectively deals with windowing issues, it also is clear that the degree of correlation between electrode sites is not computed on independent, but rather overlapping, spectral analyses.

Since the SKIL database relies exclusively on the linked ear reference, the comodulation similarity measure is strongly influenced by the fact that both sites are connected to a common source (for a review of problems with a common reference when using similarity measures see Fein, Raz, Brown, & Merrin, 1988). Nevertheless, the comodulation metric is currently being explored for possible clinical utility.

As discussed previously, there must be a balance between the number of individuals in a database and the number of variables used in assessment to account for multiple statistical tests. The SKIL database has the advantage of a large number of features (e.g., multiple conditions, single Hz bins) but has the disadvantage of a relatively small number of individuals represented in the database. This tends to increase the number of false positive findings. A solution to the problem of false positive results is to replicate findings on independent samples of data from the individual patient.

The International Brain Database

One of the most exciting developments involving qEEG database construction is the development of the first standardized International Brain Database. It overcomes the ubiquitous problems about databases that Chicurel (2000) summarized–namely that ". . . technical problems are huge, and reaching a consensus on what to archive won't be easy." A consortium of leading neuroscientists were consulted to resolve an optimal choice of tests that tap the brain's major networks and processes in the shortest amount of time. Six sites have been set up with identical equipment and software (New York, Rhode Island, London, Holland, Adelaide, and Sydney) under the auspices of a publicly listed company (The Brain Resource Company–*www.brainresource.com*), with new sites to be added progressively.

Hundreds of normative subjects have been acquired and the assessment of clinical patient groups has also recently begun. One thousand (1,000) normal controls and 1,000 patients (across the age spectrum) will be collected in the first phase.

A key dimension of this initiative (in addition to the database) is new and sophisticated analyses of EEG, ERP and autonomic activity (heart rate and electrodermal activity which are collected at the same time as the EEG/ERP). This allows not only the evaluation of state (arousal) versus trait effects, but in addition, a numerical simulation of the brain allows interpretation of EEGs according to fundamental whole brain physiological principles (in addition to simply quantifying frequency power).

Another of the most interesting new analysis methods is of 40 Hz activity (Gamma synchrony). Gamma synchrony related to cognitive processing has been observed even up to the whole brain level, and with widely separated EEG electrodes (e.g., between hemispheres). It seems, therefore, that synchrony may be an important coding mechanism across multiple scales of brain organization.

This International Brain Database involves data collection not only of EEG/ERP/autonomic in a battery of psychophysiological activation tasks, but also a comprehensive psychological test battery undertaken using a touch-screen monitor. The individual tests are listed below:

Psychological Test Battery

- Choice reaction time (speed of motor performance)
- Timing test (capacity to assess time)
- Digit span (short term memory).
- Memory Recall Test (12 words repeated 5 times with a matched distracter list after trial 4)
- Spot The Word Test (word:non-word index of IQ)
- Span of Visual Memory Test (4-second delay test of spatial short term spatial memory)
- Word Generation Test (verbal fluency test)

- Malingering Test (number recognition malingering test)
- Verbal Interference Test (test of inhibitory function)
- Switching of Attention (alternation between numbers and letters)

Psychophysiology Paradigms (NeuroScan Nuamps 40 channel/Grass electrodermal)

- Startle paradigm (fight and flight reflex)
- Go-NoGO (inhibition)
- Resting EEG (cortical stability)
- Visual tracking task (automatic tracking)
- Habituation paradigm (novelty learning)
- Auditory oddball (efficiency of target processing)
- Visual oddball (visual novelty target processing)
- Conscious and subconscious processing of facial emotions
- Visual working memory task (memory and sustained attention)
- Executive maze task (planning and error correction)

Specific event related potential measures, including P300 will be obtained. Structural and functional MRI will also be obtained for many selected individuals. Further, genetic information will be systematically collected for comparison to neuroanatomical, neurophysiological, and psychometric measures. The goal is to construct a database which can be used to integrate information directly across a variety of indices of brain structure and function.

Others

Other databases are also under development, including one using advanced EEG tomographic analysis called Low Resolution Electromagnetic Tomography (LORETA). The NovaTech EEG database currently has 84 cases and is actively adding cases. This EEG imaging technology allows for a tomographic representation of EEG sources in 3-dimensional space (see *www.NovaTechEEG.com*). This database will be useful not only in identifying deviations but approximating the location of the brain regions involved.

Hudspeth offers the NeuroRep AQR (Adult QEEG Reference Database; see *www.neurorep.com*). One of the most useful features of Hudspeth's work is the emphasis on *reliability* of measures obtained from individual patients, and the importance of EEG variability over time as a clinical index. EEG data are available for both eyes open and closed conditions. The database includes measures of absolute and relative power for 19 scalp electrodes, and all combinations (N = 171) of pair wise electrode comparisons for coherence, phase, asymmetry and correlation indices. High quality graphic representations of raw data and database comparisons also are included.

The total number of individuals in the AQR is now rather small (< 50) but additional data is being collected. Largely because of Hudspeth's extensive experience with Neurometric analysis and EEG data handling, this method can be expected to develop into an increasingly useful clinical product over time. Hudspeth (personal communication, September 14, 2002) also has presented new materials on individual patient assessment without using a database.

Frank H. Duffy, inventor and promoter of brain electrical activity mapping (BEAM; see Duffy et al., 1979), also has constructed an EEG database. This database includes both eyes-closed and eyes-open conditions, and spans a wide age range, including both children and adults. EEG data are available for 19 electrodes, and auditory and visual evoked potential measures also are included. This database was previously used in several commercial neurodiagnostic instruments (Nicolet, QSI) but to our knowledge, is not currently commercially available.

Comparison of Databases

Since QEEG databases are based on different inclusion criteria, recording methods and statistical analysis techniques, it is apparent that comparing a patient to multiple databases will likely yield different patterns of deviations. Comparing an individual to different databases confounds patient characterization with differences among the databases themselves. Therefore, we do not recommend using multiple databases in the characterization of individual patients, but rather the selection of a database that best suits the individual case.

DISCRIMINANT ANALYSIS

Both John's Neurometric analyses and Thatcher's LSNDB/Neuro-Guide include the use of discriminant analysis and clinically defined databases. The discriminant analysis is a statistical technique based on the general linear model which is used to select and weight specific variables recorded from an individual. The linear combination of these variables may be optimized so that individual patient scores are generated which correctly categorize the patient as a member of their known clinical group. When a rule is developed that successfully categorizes patients into their correct group with a high degree of accuracy, the rule is then applied to unknown individuals to see if they fit in a specific group. Neurometric analysis includes discriminant analyses for overall abnormality, learning disability, attentional disorders, alcohol abuse/ addiction, schizophrenia, depression, dementia, and head injury. However, as John has pointed out, the discriminants should only be used with individuals who have known histories of the disorders being classified. It is not legitimate to run a patient through all the discriminants to see which one "hits" and then use the hit as a diagnosis. The Thatcher LSNDB has discriminant analyses available for head injury evaluation and learning disability/hyperactivity.

There are several important issues in the use of discriminant analysis (Duffy et al., 1994). First, the discriminant attempts to classify behavioral disorders based on EEG features. It is well established that a variety of underlying patterns may be seen in seemingly homogeneous behavior disorders. Suffin and Emery (1995) have clearly demonstrated subgroups of neurometric patterns in two groups of patients with either affective or attentional disorders. Seeking invariant neurophysiological markers that are pathognomonic of complex behavioral disorders is difficult at best. If one is attempting to diagnose a learning disorder such as dyslexia, it would seem important to administer reading tests, not perform EEG discriminant analysis.

Secondly, since discriminant analyses rely on optimizing techniques, it is important to assure that a rule developed on a training set of data applies to a similarly defined test set. Without independent cross validation it is not possible to use a rule on a given individual. Even though replication by jackknifing (leave-one-out and repeat the analysis iteratively) procedures appear successful at identifying internal validity and consistency, discriminants may not yield information valuable to the treating clinician, or hold any external validity. Reports of success of discriminants often exceed 90% classification accuracy, but when used in patients with real-life comorbidities and polypharmacy, or excessive drowsiness, the techniques cannot be legitimately applied.

Further, most discriminants have been most extensively implemented as two-way classifiers. For example, a depression discriminant can only yield information on whether a patient has depression. It does not suggest that the patient is alcoholic or head injured. For these reasons, despite the apparent accuracy and reliability of certain discriminants, the discriminant analysis method has not been widely adopted in clinical practice.

CONCLUSIONS

This brief review has considered some of the important issues in construction and use of normative EEG databases, including operationalizing the concept of normalcy. Methods for recording and analysis constrain the conclusions that can be made using database comparisons. If filters are set to pass only a relatively narrow range of EEG frequencies, no statements can be made about the frequencies filtered out and lost to subsequent analyses. If broad bands are used, important deviations appearing at single frequencies or a restricted range of frequencies will be missed.

A critical concern is the number of variables in a database relative to the number of cases along with the problem of multiple statistical testing. Most databases contain an unfavorable variables/cases ratio and replication of findings should be strongly encouraged in order to limit false positive results. As databases grow to incorporate more recording electrodes, frequency bands, and task conditions the problem of false positive findings is more relevant.

The importance of the recording electrode and the need for remontaging norms has been emphasized. The linked ear reference is a particularly poor choice of references since it can be both active and asymmetric, yet historically it has been the default reference for most databases. Use of multiple references is suggested to minimize the bias inherent in use of a single reference point.

A brief review of the characteristics of several major databases is presented. Each has advantages and disadvantages but newer databases will exploit new technological developments and increasing sophistication in statistical analysis of EEG data. Implementing new measures such as variability over time and extraction of features such as event-related desynchronization (see Pfurtscheller, Maresch, & Schuy, 1985) and gamma synchrony (Rennie, Wright, & Robinson, 2000) are likely to have important clinical impact. Caution is urged in the use of automated classification by discriminant analysis.

REFERENCES

Ahn, H., Prichep, L. S., John, E. R., Baird, H., Trepetin, M., & Kaye, H. (1980). Developmental equations reflect brain dysfunctions. *Science, 210*, 1259-1261.

Chicurel, M. (2000). Databasing the brain. *Nature, 406*, 822-825.

Donchin, E. (1987). The P300 as a metric for mental workload. *Electroencephalography and Clinical Neurophysiology, 39* (Suppl.), 338-343.

Duffy, F. H., Burchfiel, J. L., & Lombroso, C. T. (1979). Brain electrical activity mapping (BEAM): A method for extending the clinical utility of EEG and evoked potential data. *Annals of Neurology, 5* (4), 309-321.

Duffy, F. H., Hughes, J. R., Miranda, F., Bernad, P., & Cook, P. (1994). Status of quantitative EEG (QEEG) in clinical practice. *Clinical Electroencephalography, 25* (4), VI-XXII.

Fein, G., Raz, J., Brown F. F., & Merrin, E. L. (1988). Common reference coherence data are confounded by power and phase effects. *Electroencephalography and Clinical Neurophysiology, 69* (6), 581-584.

Gunkelman, J. (2000). Hjorth referencing in QEEG. *Journal of Neurotherapy, 4* (1), 57-62.

Hammond, D. C., & Gunkelman, J. (2001). *The art of artifacting.* Salt Lake City, Utah: Society for Neuronal Regulation (see *www.snr-jnt.org*).

John, E. R., Karmel, B. Z., Corning, W. C., Easton, P., Brown, D., Ahn, H. et al. 1977. Neurometrics: Numerical taxonomy identifies different profiles of brain functions within groups of behaviorally similar people. *Science, 196,* 1393-1410.

John, E. R., Prichep, L., Ahn, H., Easton, P., Fridman, J., & Kaye, H. (1983). Neurometric evaluation of cognitive dysfunctions and neurological disorders in children. *Progress in Neurobiology, 21* (4), 239-290.

John, E. R., Prichep, L. S., & Easton, P. (1987). Normative data banks and neurometrics. Basic concepts, methods, results of norm construction. In A. S. Gevins & A. Remond (Eds.), *Methods of analysis of brain electrical and magnetic signals* (pp. 449-495). Amsterdam: Elsevier.

Johnstone, J. (2002). Bispectral analysis of the EEG: A brief technical note. *Journal of Neurotherapy, 6* (3), 77-81.

Lorensen, T., & Dickson, P. (2002). Quantitative EEG normative databases: A comparative investigation [Abstract]. *Journal of Neurotherapy, 6* (1), 89-90.

Misulis, K. E., & Fakhoury, T. (2001). *Spehlmann's evoked potential primer* (3rd ed.). Philadelphia: Elsevier (Butterworth-Heinemann).

Niedermeyer, E., & Lopes da Silva, F. (Eds.). (1999). *Electroencephalography: Basic principles, clinical applications, and related fields* (4th ed.). Baltimore: Lippincott, Williams & Wilkins.

Pfurtscheller, G., Maresch, H., & Schuy, S. (1985). ERD (event-related desynchronization) mapping: A new procedure for functional brain diagnosis. *Biomedical Technology (Berlin), 3* (1-2), 2-6.

Rennie C. J., Wright, J. J., & Robinson P. A. (2000). Mechanisms of cortical electrical activation and emergence of gamma rhythm. *Journal of Theoretical Biology, 205* (1), 17-35.

Scherg, M., Ille, N., Bornfleth, H., & Berg, P. (2002). Advanced tools for digital EEG review: Virtual source montages, whole-head mapping, correlation, and phase analysis. *Journal of Clinical Neurophysiology, 19* (2), 91-112.

Sigl J. C., & Chamoun N. C. (1994). An introduction to bispectral analysis for the EEG. *Journal of Clinical Monitoring, 10,* 392-404.

Sterman, M. B., & Kaiser, D. (2001). Comodulation: A new qEEG analysis metric for assessment of structural and functional disorders of the central nervous system. *Journal of Neurotherapy, 4* (3), 73-83.

Suffin, S. C., & Emory, W. H. (1995). Neurometric subgroups in attentional and affective disorders and their association with pharmacotherapeutic outcome. *Clinical Electroencephalography, 26*, 76-83.

Thatcher, R. W. (1998). EEG normative databases and EEG biofeedback. *Journal of Neurotherapy, 2* (4), 8-39.

Tyner, F., & Knott, J. (1983). *Fundamentals of EEG technology Vol. 1*. New York: Raven Press.

Quantitative EEG Normative Databases:
A Comparative Investigation

Tamara D. Lorensen, BSc Grad Dip
Paul Dickson, BSocSc Bpsych

SUMMARY. *Introduction.* No clearly defined or universally accepted standards exist which practitioners and researchers can use to determine which quantitative electroencephalographic (QEEG) database is suitable to their needs. Diverse computational and methodological approaches across QEEG databases have been vigorously defended by their respective proponents and commonly misunderstood by practitioners. The purpose of this paper is to facilitate widespread discussion from which a universal set of standards can be agreed upon and applied to QEEG databases.

Method. A broad set of criteria was developed from an extensive liter-

Tamara D. Lorensen is affiliated with the School of Health, Faculty of Psychology and Counseling, Queensland University of Technology, and the Neurotherapy Centre, Queensland, Australia.

Paul Dickson is affiliated with the Neurotherapy Centre, Queensland, Australia.

Address correspondence to: Tamara D. Lorensen, P.O. Box 144, Kelvin Grove DC, Queensland 4059, Australia (E-mail: tamara@tpgi.com.au).

The authors wish to acknowledge the contributions of M. Barry Sterman, PhD to this paper. Dr. Sterman graciously read this paper and made a number of suggestions regarding the form and the content of the paper, which were incorporated. It should be noted that Dr. Sterman is the co-author of the SKIL database, one of the databases considered in this paper.

ature review and included issues of sampling, acquisition, hardware/ software, control of confounding variables, and additional issues associated with disclosure, accessibility, and the screening of potential users. These criteria were then applied to the Hudspeth, John, Sterman-Kaiser, and Thatcher databases.

Results. Results revealed reasonable concordance in data acquisition methods despite departures in inclusion/exclusion criteria and sample sizes. Significant differences were apparent in the controls used for possible confounding variables and the relative importance given to these variables.

Conclusions. Research, clinical, and ethical implications are discussed, and it is recommended that the QEEG scientific community establish peer-review procedures and processes which prevent database manufacturers from seducing peers and clinicians with technocratic information and techniques that appear to confuse the user or oversimplify the complexity and richness of QEEG applications. *[Article copies available for a fee from The Haworth Document Delivery Service: 1-800-HAWORTH. E-mail address: <docdelivery@haworthpress.com> Website: <http://www. HaworthPress.com> © 2003 by The Haworth Press, Inc. All rights reserved.]*

KEYWORDS. Quantitative electroencephalogram, QEEG, QEEG database, normative methodology, methods, standards, controversy

INTRODUCTION

Through examination of electroencephalographic (EEG) phenomena, researchers have sought to investigate a diversity of brain related issues ranging from sleep and epilepsy to head injury and attention deficit disorder. This research has promoted the development and publication of a substantial body of literature. Historically, the literature has been based almost exclusively upon qualitative visual evaluations of the clinical EEG (Duffy, McAnulty, Jones, Als, & Albert, 1993). Researchers have used the outcomes of clinical EEG visual inspection to assist in developing working hypotheses that have aided in the formulation of more accurate diagnoses in a number of research areas (Duffy, Hughes, Miranda, Bernad, & Cook, 1994). Another objective of visual examination has been to screen the background composition of the EEG for spatial distribution of frequencies and temporal stability of various frequencies (Duffy, Jensen, Erba, Burchfiel, & Lombroso, 1984). While neurological diseases that produce focal or paroxysmal abnormal EEG

stand out visibly against the background spectra, challenges have occurred in identifying various frequency compositions over time by mere
visual inspection alone (Duffy, 1989).

Development of computer technology accompanied a new era of research capabilities that made it possible for investigators to examine
EEG patterns using quantitative analytical methods (John, 1989; Kaiser, 2000; Sterman, 2001). The development of quantitative EEG analysis has afforded researchers the opportunity to scientifically investigate
whether large samples of participants who meet medical and psychological criteria for normality also display stable, reliable and common
patterns in their EEG. Similarly, other researchers also began to consider whether groups of participants with varying psychological disorders also displayed unique EEG patterns that were distinct from the
EEG patterns of the non-clinical population samples. Some of the research that has compared the EEG patterns of non-clinical controls and
clinical subjects, separated on the basis of either medical or psychological criteria, demonstrated that there are clear, valid and reliable distinc-
tions in the characteristics of the EEG across groups (John, Prichep,
Fridman, & Easton, 1988; John, 1989). The implication of this research
is that certain EEG patterns can be common and unique to both non-
clinical and clinical groups of subjects.

While John (1989) argued that there were clear benefits in using
quantitative electroencephalography (QEEG) to discriminate between
certain populations, Fisch and Pedley (1989) retained fervent reserva-
tions about the reliability and validity of various QEEG measures.
Some of the concerns expressed were centered upon the type of instru-
mentation and acquisition devices used, the data reduction methods employed, and the normative databases used to compare non-clinical and
clinical populations. Additional concerns have been consistently voiced
about the methodological standards and related efficacy of QEEG analyses (American Psychiatric Association Task Force, 1991; Duffy et al.,
1994; Oken & Chiappa, 1986; Veldhuizen, Jonkman, & Poorvliet, 1993).
Kaiser (2000) suggests that as yet no adequate methodological standards appropriate to QEEG analysis have been adopted within the field.
This could be a significant factor underlying any erroneous results arising from QEEG (Kaiser, 2000). According to Kaiser (2000) studies
have shown that similar methodological approaches have achieved reliable outcomes based on QEEG analyses.

Likewise in a recent review by Hughes and John (1999) the authors
suggested that the state of QEEG in the last decade has shown itself to
remain highly reliable. Hughes and John proposed that the electrical ac-

tivity of the brain is homeostatically regulated, and that this results in a predictable frequency composition of the background EEG.

In recent years, a keen interest has developed in more widespread use of the QEEG, particularly in applied clinical settings. Where QEEG technology was once the domain of established research settings and university laboratories, QEEG analysis is now available at the grass roots level in clinical settings. Consequently, the plethora of methodological issues surrounding QEEG is particularly relevant. Some practitioners, preferring to rely on QEEG data to inform certain components of their clinical practice such as evaluation and neurofeedback applications, commonly choose to select one database to meet all their clinical needs. Furthermore, there are practitioners who use additional services provided by certain databases such as discrimination, diagnosis, evaluation, interpretation and reporting of client status. Consequently, those practitioners face the added difficulty of evaluating the accuracy of these interpretations, assuming they evaluate these services at all.

This review highlights some key issues that make a compelling case for the urgent commencement of an applied and ongoing evaluation of QEEG normative databases. The major aim of this paper is to facilitate discussion and encourage ongoing appraisal of some of the current databases. This will be achieved by applying a number of criteria proposed by other authors in the field (Fisch & Pedley, 1989; John, Prichep, & Easton, 1987; Kaiser, 2000) to compare and evaluate several QEEG databases. These criteria will be used to draw attention to methodological issues that need further disclosure or additional clarification. A likely result is the application of greater scientific rigor by both practitioners and new researchers.

METHOD

The research conducted for this paper was both inductive and exploratory. At the outset, a literature search was made for several authors who were known to have developed normative databases. Searches began with published peer-reviewed articles across a variety of journals and accessed via Queensland University Library databases. The journal searches included the *Annals of Neurology, Biological Psychiatry, Clinical Electroencephalography, Electroencephalography and Clinical Neurophysiology, Journal of Clinical Psychiatry, Journal of Neuropsychiatry and Clinical Neurosciences, Journal of Neurotherapy* and *Psychiatry Research.*

Where the data were unavailable from these sources, electronic on-line searches for authors, subjects, and commercial normative databases were conducted using internet search engines. The normative databases examined were John (NxLink, 2001); Hudspeth (Hudspeth, 1999); Sterman-Kaiser (Sterman-Kaiser Imaging Laboratory, 2000) and Thatcher (Thatcher, Biver, Walker, North, & Curtin, 2000). The John database is particularly large and this proved to be an obstacle in accessing information. This investigation only examined the studies reported in John et al. (1987). It is our understanding that the databases examined are in constant review and development, which influenced the currency of our information.

The criteria used and displayed in Table 1 were drawn from the following published works: American Psychiatric Association Task Force, 1991; Duffy et al., 1994; John et al., 1987; Kaiser, 2000, 2001; Kaiser & Sterman, 1994; Pollock & Schneider, 1990; Thatcher, 1998. These works showed agreement in terms of the issues raised regarding standards of QEEG methodology.

Table 1 provides a summary of the participants and normality criteria. Details of sampling or recruitment were not clearly addressed by the database developers. This made it difficult to evaluate how well sound

TABLE 1. Sampling Subject Characteristics of Participants and Normality Criteria

	Hudspeth	John study 2	John study 1	Sterman-Kaiser	Thatcher
Participants Size (N)	31	120	386	135	625
Age range	NS	17-90	6-90	18-55	2 mths-83
(Children)	0	0	306	0	470
(Adults)	31	120	80	135	155
Gender	NS	63 M 57 F	NS	80% M 20% F	56.8% M 43.2% F
Normality Criteria	Interview questionnaire LNNB	Type not specified	NS adults elsewhere children	Questionnaire (appended in software manual) Oldfield Handedness	Interview questionnaire WAIS WISC and further tests

NS = Not Specified

experimental protocols had been followed throughout this stage of data collection.

The exclusion and inclusion criteria used to screen for normality were also examined. It is generally accepted among researchers that the appropriate application of well developed and relevant screening procedures promotes homogeneity of the sample being investigated (Pollock & Schneider, 1990). It is evident that there is significant variation in the size of the samples used, the age ranges reported, the percentage split between males and females and the normality criteria used. A summary of the inclusion/exclusion criteria used in each database is included below.

Hudspeth

An interview and questionnaire

An uneventful prenatal, perinatal and postnatal period

No disorders of consciousness

No reported head injuries

No history of central nervous system diseases, convulsions or seizures due to any cause

No abnormal deviation with regard to mental and physical development

No reported substance or drug abuse

Neuropsychological Testing:

Luria-Nebraska Neuropsychological battery

Met standard criteria for normality including Pathognomicity T >70

No more than three clinical scales with T > 70

John

Study 1:   John reports that the criteria for normality and details of processing were to be found in other literature. Investigation of this revealed that this reference was for children only and the information pertaining to adults was not found.

Study 2:   Self-supporting evidence

Functioning in job/household related activities

No history of head injury with loss of consciousness

No history of EEG abnormality or neurological disorders

No current prescription medications (except anti-hypertensive)

No history of drug/alcohol abuse

No subjective complaints of cognitive dysfunction

IQ estimates were in the normal range

Sterman-Kaiser

Students and lab personal (50%)

Recruited volunteers from the community (25%)

Air Force personnel including pilots, ground crew and administrative personnel (25%)

All subjects completed a handedness inventory

A questionnaire was used to screen for medical history and drug use

Recent life events (appended in accompanying manual)

The Air Force personnel used (25%) were intensively pre-screened as a condition of their service and were subject to regular medical exams and unusually high levels of drug use scrutiny.

Thatcher

Thatcher does not specify who received the testing or the different tests administered to adults or children but does report:

An uneventful prenatal, perinatal and postnatal period

No disorders of consciousness

No history of central nervous diseases

No convulsions either febrile or psychogenic

No abnormal deviation with regard to mental and physical development

Neuropsychological Testing:

Weschler Adult Intelligence Scale (WAIS) 17-adult

Weschler Intelligence Scale Children (WISC) 6-16.99 years

Other Tests

Agpar score

Vineland Social Maturity

2-3.99 yrs. McCarthy Intelligence Scale

4-5.99 yrs. Weschler pre-school & primary scale intelligence

WRAT

Grade cards from the school system

Peg board of skilled motor movements

MIT

Eight item laterality test

Hollingshead four factors of social status

Presence of environmental toxins (children only)

Table 2 contains a summary of the acquisition procedures used in database development. The development and implementation of standardized procedures in acquiring QEEG data ensures that subjects are treated in a similar fashion during all stages of data acquisition. Some authors have detailed these issues and identified the need to hold features in the environment constant. Recommendations have been made to record in the same room, use the same technician, use the same acquisition instruments, and standardize recording techniques and procedures (John et al., 1987; Kaiser, 2000). John et al. (1987, p. 453) emphatically states that " . . . in order to construct useful normative databanks . . . procedures must be meticulously standardized and precisely described." However, it appears that several of the more expansive databases were combined from disparate facilities where standardization of populations and collection methods were difficult to confirm.

Electrophysiological Procedure

All databases report similar approaches to procedures such as linked ears reference and the use of the 10/20 montage. However, there is evi-

TABLE 2. Summary of Acquisition Procedures Relating to Hardware and Software

Acquisition Hardware	Hudspeth	John study 1 & 2	Sterman-Kaiser	Thatcher
Reference	Linked ears	Linked ears	Linked ears	Linked ears
Montage	10/20	10/20	10/20	10/20
Impedance	3 K ohms	NS	5 K ohms	5 K ohms 10 K ohms
Electrodes	19 2 EOG	19	19	16 1 bipolar EOG
Acquisition Software				
Condition	Eyes closed Eyes open	Eyes closed Eyes open	Eyes closed Eyes open Task Task	Eyes closed Eyes open
Record duration	60 secs Artifact free	30-60 secs Artifact free	2-4 mins	60 secs Artifact free
Band widths	Single Hz Delta 0.5-3.5 Theta 3.5-7 Alpha 7-13 Beta 13-22	Delta 1.5-3.5 Theta 3.5-7.5 Alpha 7.5-12.5 Beta 12.5-25	Single Hz User defined Delta 1-3 Theta 3-7 Alpha 7-12 Beta 12-15 Beta 15-20	Delta 0-2 Theta 3.5-7 Alpha 7-13 Beta 13-22
Artifact method	On-line Visual	Automatic Visual	Automatic Visual State transition	Automatic Visual

NS = Not Specified

dence that other procedures were not as well standardized across databases. In particular, while nineteen channels were used for recording by three of the four databases, in the Thatcher database the montage appears to be comprised of only 16 channels, omitting the mid-line sites (Thatcher et al., 2000). It is also evident from Table 2 that the Thatcher database differs from the other databases in terms of the consistency in the level of impedance that was accepted. Thatcher reports that most of the impedance measures were less than 5 K ohms, but he does not provide specific details pertaining to the number of impedance measurements recorded which were below 5 K ohms and the number of impedance measures that were recorded between 5 K ohms and 10 K ohms.

Other areas of variation across databases were also evident. For example, only two of the four databases reported using ElectroOculogram (EOG) leads. Sterman-Kaiser also disclosed additional information not apparent from the other databases. In the Sterman-Kaiser database the EEG data recorded were subjected to 2 Hz high pass and 30 Hz low pass filters, with roll-offs of 12 and 48 dB/octave, respectively. It is specified that data were digitized at 128 samples per second. John reports time epochs of 256 sample values at a digitization rate of 100 Hz. This was also reported in the Hudspeth and Thatcher databases. Technical texts report that these factors play a role in the acquisition and evaluation of EEG data and it is important that these details are more completely reported in the future.

In terms of recording procedures, there was further evidence of variation across databases. Three databases recorded eyes-open and eyes-closed conditions only; whereas Sterman-Kaiser adds two cognitive task conditions to the data acquisition. They also limit recording length to three to four minutes, with two to four replications of each state. John reports including 60 seconds of artifact free data (or a minimum of 30 seconds of artifact free data) with a single replication in the eyes-closed condition only. Pollock and Schneider (1990) report three to five minutes of EEG acquisition under the eyes-closed, resting condition might be optimal due to the high level of variation in a subject's level of consciousness during more prolonged recordings. It is evident that there are differences of opinion about what is optimal in the length of the record and the reported length of record used in data analysis. However a key factor is homogeneity of state during recording.

Table 2 also shows that the bandwidths used varied across databases. While John and Thatcher used standard bandwidths, both Sterman-Kaiser and Hudspeth provide users with the ability to analyze single hertz bins and both of these databases offer unique data reduction capabilities not present on other systems. Some researchers now suggest that standard bands are an outdated concept. Researchers have never agreed upon standard band cutoffs and even a cursory review of the literature shows that the bandwidths used are highly variable (Duffy et al., 1984; Kaiser, 2001; Pollock & Schneider, 1990). Despite differences of opinion regarding this issue, it is logical that such variations in bandwidths affect the sensitivity of EEG measures and their comparability. This provides additional justification for the adoption of either single hertz bins or standardized bandwidths in the future development of databases.

Artifact rejection techniques were found to be similar across databases. For three databases artifact rejection occurs online and epochs are excluded if the voltage exceeds a pre-set limit. Sterman-Kaiser use wavelet analysis for estimating the period of data corruption from artifact in off-line correction. Sterman-Kaiser also provides the rationale and supporting evidence for excluding the initial 30 seconds of data due to state transition effects.

A variety of methods used to control for confounding variables were disclosed by the databases. Two issues have been targeted which we believe are worth specific consideration at this time in the genesis of normative EEG: time of day and state conditions. Table 3 provides an overview of the way the databases addressed these issues and it appears evident that these issues were only addressed in the Sterman-Kaiser database. The Thatcher database reported using randomization to control for time-of-day effects, but the methods used to achieve randomization were not disclosed and it could be inferred that any randomization was done ex-post facto in an attempt to offset less than optimal control procedures.

The SKIL database reports that it was able to obtain sufficient data to allow for the analysis of time-of-day effects. Each subject provided two to four replications of each recording condition across several time periods. These data generated a combination of cross-sectional and longitudinal outcomes over varying time categories to evaluate diurnal influences on EEG characteristics. Data provided twenty-one time-of-day categories using 274 eyes-closed and 274 eyes-open conditions. Each category was spaced in one-hour intervals every half hour. The number of subjects in each interval ranged from 15 to 19 in the 9:00 a.m. to noon intervals and 29 to 38 in the noon to 5:00 p.m. intervals. Subjects were not sampled more than once in each time interval. It was found that the active task conditions did not require time-of-day corrections. It is apparent that this variable has been contentious in its reported

TABLE 3. Summary of Two Criteria and Treatment of Confounding Variables

Controlled Variables	Hudspeth	John study 1 & 2	Sterman	Thatcher
Time-of-day	NS	NS	Specified	Random
State transitions	NS	NS	Initial 30 sec. deleted	NS

NS = Not Specified

effects on the EEG. However, Sterman and Kaiser (Sterman-Kaiser Imaging Laboratory, 2000) have provided the rationale for its inclusion together with supporting evidence from the chronobiology literature. According to Kaiser and Sterman (1994) this evidence exists and it may be optimal to include diurnal effects in a well-designed database.

The efficacy in examining task conditions in EEG spectral parameters has also been demonstrated particularly between rest and several cognitive tasks (Fernandez et al., 1994). Increasing interest in the EEG of disorders of attention indicate the need for inclusion of recording cognitive task conditions (Sterman, Kaiser, & Veigel, 1996; Sterman, 1999, 2000). This is another issue that needs to be addressed and it seems that future research and the development of specific task conditions for inclusion in each of the databases is justified.

Table 4 presents some other issues that we considered relevant in reviewing the literature. The result of extensive searches indicated that the procedures and methodology were more difficult to access for some databases than others. Specifically it was difficult to access the sample size, and a description of the normative sample used in the John database. In contrast, other database providers have this information readily available. We found that Sterman-Kaiser and Thatcher made access easy via online searches.

It would be useful for database owners to screen potential users of their databases. A potential source of unexamined variability is the lack of quality control of the clinicians who can gain access to databases. Further, there is no evidence that minimum standards of technical expertise are imposed on practitioners prior to gaining access to the data-

TABLE 4. Identified Issues of Further Concern Relating to Information Accessibility, Screening of Users and Clarity of Communication

	Hudspeth	John study 1 & 2	Sterman-Kaiser	Thatcher
Accessibility and reporting of database description	Easy	Difficult	Easy	Easy
Screening of potential users of databases such as clinicians and researchers	NS	NS	Training for new users	NS
Expression of ideas and demonstrably clear communication to the reader	Average	Challenging	Average	Average

NS = Not Specified

base services. To date, there are no set standards such as a minimum number of courses or hours of training that database owners require practitioners to complete. It is our contention that minimum levels of experience need to be acquired and ongoing training needs to be provided for people using the databases. It is also our understanding that Sterman-Kaiser require attendance at introductory and advanced training courses prior to the purchase of the software for new users.

The statistical methods used to handle the large data sets generated by EEG acquisition are complex and retain hidden assumptions. There is significant disagreement among expert statisticians over the interpretation and suitability of statistical techniques used in QEEG. We are exposed daily to conclusions based on sophisticated inferential statistical reasoning which for many is tedious and difficult.

Concerns with statistical issues have been expressed by Oken and Chiappa (1986). They suggest that statisticians review papers to prevent statistically unsophisticated readers from being exposed to papers that may contain erroneous, invalidated and chance results and conclusions. Furthermore the scientific community is responsible for preventing readers from being 'seduced' by certain techniques that may appear to be able to objectify diagnoses or evaluations. A. K. Ashbury, Editor of the *Annals of Neurology*, publisher of the Oken and Chiappa paper, added an editorial comment suggesting that even among experts there are fundamental disagreements and that for many of us statistics are obscure.

DISCUSSION

With recent advancements in computer technology the capacity to acquire real-time neurophysiology data has grown exponentially. Our intention in this article has been to draw attention to some of the issues that have emerged from this rapid growth. In particular, we have highlighted some of the differences that need to be identified and scrutinized within the normative EEG database field. Areas are identified where improvements can be made in the services provided by these databases. It is hoped that this article creates a greater interest in standardizing methodologies and reporting procedures. The failure to do so creates a continued risk of justifiable criticism by other professional industries (American Psychiatric Association Task Force, 1991). As Duffy et al. (1994) state, there is no agreed upon standard QEEG test battery or analytical process, and while this statement was made some years ago, it is our impression that there has not been much change.

The implications of this article also extend to the provision of easily understood information for practitioners. How the database owners address the issues raised in this paper and whether in the future the databases will be used more appropriately by practitioners and researchers is still to be determined. More specifically, it is important that the issue of the inappropriate use of databases be addressed and rectified through training.

Concurrently, there is the challenge of characterizing the limits of normal EEG biologic variability and the ability to distinguish this from pathological brain function. This is particularly applicable to controlling for variables such as time-of-day (Fisch & Pedley, 1989) or the use of arbitrary standard bandwidths vs. individualized custom bands. Additionally, proponents of the databases, including the developers themselves, should consider that financial or academic interests in promoting their own database could impact how their work is viewed. This reality further highlights the need for accurate, scientifically rigorous reporting and review. Reporting which is insufficient or which fails to highlight the complexities associated with the EEG signal and with its quantitative analysis misleads practitioners and the decisions they must make about their clients' treatment.

Critical to this analysis is the recognition that databases have in fact been developed over many years. Some of the differences noted seem to be a reflection of time-line development, and illustrate the importance of matching and updating database development to reflect current QEEG research.

Finally, the implications of this research identify a need to further refine existing methods and principles in order to truly develop the potentially broad ranging clinical utility of the QEEG. One requirement is to demonstrate the validity and reliability of all QEEG databases through peer-reviewed published studies. Further, it should be recognized that data cannot be combined or compared if different methods and standards are used. Even use of the same database across various studies with differences in methodology risks invalidation of the findings. The practitioner should not overlook these considerations. Nevertheless, the QEEG database has proven to be an efficacious tool that has expanded our understanding of the brain, of behavior, and of the objectives of neurotherapy.

REFERENCES

American Psychiatric Association Task Force (1991). Quantitative electroencephalography: A report on the present state of computerized EEG techniques. *American Journal of Psychiatry, 148* (7), 961-964.

Cacot, P., Tesolin, B., & Sebban, C. (1995). Diurnal variations of EEG power in healthy adults. *Electroencephalography and Clinical Neurophysiology, 94,* 305-312.

Duffy, F. H. (1989). Brain electrical activity mapping: Clinical applications. *Psychiatry Research, 29,* 379-384.

Duffy, F. H., Hughes, J. R., Miranda, F., Bernad, P., & Cook, P. (1994). Status of quantitative EEG (QEEG) in clinical practice. *Clinical Electroencephalography, 25* (4), VI-XXII.

Duffy, F. H., Jensen, F., Erba, G., Burchfiel, J. L., & Lombroso, C. T. (1984). Extraction of clinical information from electroencephalographic background activity: The combined use of brain electrical activity mapping and intravenous sodium thiopental. *Annals of Neurology, 15* (1), 22-30.

Duffy, F. H., McAnulty, G. B., Jones, K., Als, H., & Albert, M. (1993). Brain electrical correlates of psychological measures: Strategies and problems. *Brain Topography, 5* (4), 399-412.

Fernandez, T., Harmony, T., Rodriguez, M., Bernal, J., Silva, J., Reyes, A. et al. (1994). EEG activation patterns during the performance of tasks involving different components of mental calculation. *Electroencephalography and Clinical Neurophysiology, 94,* 175-182.

Fisch, B. J., & Pedley, T. A. (1989). The role of quantitative topographic mapping or 'Neurometrics' in the diagnosis of psychiatric and neurological disorders: The cons. *Electroencephalography and Clinical Neurophysiology, 73,* 5-9.

Hudspeth, W. J. (1999). NeuroRep QEEG Analysis and Report System, (Version 4.0) [Computer software]. Los Osos, CA: Grey Matter Inc.

John, E. R. (1989). The role of quantitative EEG topographic mapping or 'Neurometrics' in the diagnosis of psychiatric and neurological disorders: The pros. *Electroencephalography and Clinical Neurophysiology, 73,* 2-4.

John, E. R., Prichep, L. S., & Easton, P. (1987). Normative data banks and Neurometrics. Basic concepts, methods and results of norm constructions. In A. S. Gevins & A. Remond (Eds.), *Handbook of electroencephalography and clinical neurophysiology. Revised Series.* (Vol. 1, pp. 449-495). Amsterdam: Elsevier.

John, E. R., Prichep, L., Fridman, J., & Easton, P. (1988). Neurometrics: Computer-assisted differential diagnosis of brain dysfunction. *Science, 239,* 162-169.

Kaiser, D. A. (2000). QEEG: State of the art, or state of confusion. *Journal of Neurotherapy, 4* (2), 57-75.

Kaiser, D. A. (2001). Rethinking standard bands. *Journal of Neurotherapy, 5* (1-2), 87-96.

Kaiser, D. A., & Sterman, M. B. (1994). *Periodicity of standardized EEG spectral measures across the waking day.* Retrieved July 17, 2001, from *http://www.skiltopo.com/papers/kaiser94.htm*

NxLink. (2001). *Neurometric analysis system.* Richland, WA: NxLink Ltd.

Oken, B. S., & Chiappa, K. H. (1986). Statistical issues concerning computerized analysis of brainwave topography. *Annals of Neurology, 19* (5), 493-494.

Pollock.V. E., & Schneider, L. S. (1990). Quantitative waking EEG research on depression. *Biological Psychiatry, 27,* 757-780.

Sterman, M. B. (1999). Functional patterns and their physiological origins in the waking EEG: A theoretical integration with implications for event-related EEG responses. In G. Pfurtscheller & F. H. Lopes da Silva (Eds.), *Handbook of electroencephalography and clinical neurophysiology. Revised Series* (Vol. 6, pp. 233-242). Amsterdam: Elsevier.

Sterman, M. B. (2000). EEG markers for attention deficit disorder: Pharmacological and neurofeedback applications. *Child Study Journal, 30.* 1-23.

Sterman, M. B. (2001). Comodulation: A new QEEG analysis metric for assessment of structural and functional disorders of the CNS. *Journal of Neurotherapy, 4* (3), 73-83.

Sterman-Kaiser Imaging Laboratory. (2000). SKIL Topometric Software Manual Version 2.05. Los Angeles: Sterman-Kaiser Imaging Laboratory.

Sterman, M. B., Kaiser, D. A., & Veigel, B. (1996). Spectral analysis of event-related EEG responses during short-term memory performance. *Brain Topography, 9* (1), 21-30.

Thatcher, R. W. (1998). Normative EEG databases and EEG biofeedback. *Journal of Neurotherapy, 2* (4), 8-39.

Thatcher, R. W., Biver, C. J., Walker, R. A., North, D. M., & Curtin, B. S. (2000). *Thatcher EEG normative database.* Retrieved July, 17, 2001 from *http://www.appliedneuroscience.com*

Veldhuizen, R. J., Jonkman, E. J., & Poorvliet, D. C. J. (1993). Sex differences in age regression parameters of healthy adults-normative data and practical implications. *Electroencephalography and Clinical Neurophysiology, 86,* 377-384.

Databases or Specific Training Protocols for Neurotherapy? A Proposal for a "Clinical Approach to Neurotherapy"

Jaime Romano-Micha, MD

SUMMARY. This paper reviews and summarizes the use of quantitative electroencephalography (EEG) and normative databases in the design and application of EEG biofeedback (neurotherapy) for clinical purposes. It is argued that such a statistical approach to EEG analysis ignores important individual patient data observed in the raw EEG.

While databases provide important information for understanding brain function, they have important limitations for patient diagnosis and as guides to the training of brain waves. On the other hand, although the use of specific training protocols and the training of specific electroencephalographic frequencies have been shown to be useful in improv-

Jaime Romano-Micha is Clinical Neurophysiologist and Director, Centro Neuro Psico Pedagogico S. C. (www.cnpp.org.mx).

Address correspondence to: Dr. Jaime Romano-Micha, Gral. Leon # 38, Col. San Miguel Chapultepec, Mexico City, 11850, Mexico (E-mail: jromano@cnpp.org.mx).

The author wants to thank T. J. La Vaque for his valuable comments regarding this article and Darlene Nelson for editorial assistance.

The brain maps in Figures 2, 3, and 4 were obtained by the use of EEGC software developed by Dr. Jaime Romano-Micha (www.eegmapping.com).

ing symptoms in different neurological and psychological disorders, they are insufficient to structure a rational neurofeedback training protocol.

It is assumed that neurotherapy produces fundamental changes in brain function. Although there have been no published reports to date of iatrogenic problems arising from neurotherapy, the potential for such problems raises ethical concerns the individual practitioner should consider. In this paper the advantages and limitations of databases and the use of specific training protocols are discussed, and a "clinical approach" for neurotherapy is proposed. *[Article copies available for a fee from The Haworth Document Delivery Service: 1-800-HAWORTH. E-mail address: <docdelivery@haworthpress.com> Website: <http://www.HaworthPress.com> © 2003 by The Haworth Press, Inc. All rights reserved.]*

KEYWORDS. Brain mapping, neurofeedback, EEG databases, neurotherapy, qEEG, clinical approach to neurotherapy, neurofeedback training protocols

INTRODUCTION

Neurofeedback and brain mapping represent two related new fields in neuroscience (Romano-Micha, 2000). Their evolution in the last two decades has been possible due to technological developments and more specifically to the increased power of computers used in the fields of neurophysiology and psychophysiology. As in any new field of knowledge, neurofeedback and brain mapping are going through different stages of development. At present, neurofeedback is in a stage of growth and maturation. With time, cumulative experience, and verification via clinical and research data, the strengths and weaknesses of neurofeedback will be identified. Thereafter it will assume its proper place as both a research and clinical tool for various applications.

NEUROFEEDBACK

Neurofeedback began in the late 1960s, when Kamiya (1968) reported that it was possible to voluntarily control alpha waves. Other investigators (Beaty, Greenberg, Deibler, & O'Hanlon, 1974) implemented further experiments on theta waves, evoked cortical responses, and EEG phase synchrony in specialized learning processes. More experiments followed, with specific rhythms such as the sensorimotor rhythm (SMR) emerging as having therapeutic effects in epilepsy (Sterman, 1972) and in patients with attention deficit disorders (Lubar, 1991).

Since then, there have been an increasing number of different training protocols for specific frequencies and frequency ratios and success reported in treating a wide variety of disorders such as addictive behaviors (Ochs, 1992; Rosenfeld, 1992; Peniston & Kulkosky, 1989), affective disorders (Rosenfeld, 1997) and stroke rehabilitation (Rozelle & Budzynski, 1995) among others.

NEUROPHYSIOLOGY

Electroencephalography (EEG) as one of the neurophysiological techniques has its own history, starting in the early 1920s. Electroencephalography has evolved tremendously since the time in 1924 when Hans Berger was able to record an electric signal from his son's brain for the first time. Berger was obsessed with trying to find material events (electrical brain potentials) that were related to mental phenomena, in which he included telepathy. Although he did not accomplish his final goal, he was able to establish the fundamentals necessary for the development of a powerful instrument for analysis of the cerebral cortical function (Berger, 1969).

Since then and with the use of powerful computer techniques for signal analysis–such as Fourier analysis–the era of quantitative EEG began. Grass and Gibbs (1938), Walter (1963), and Bickford, Brimm, Berger, and Aung (1973) were among the investigators who pioneered the area of computerized EEG.

With sophisticated visual representation of this analyzed signal, starting with the Compressed Spectral Array designed by Bickford and later as brain maps with the use of mathematical algorithms such as linear, Laplacian or quadratic interpolations, it was possible to increase the capacity of the EEG to characterize more precisely some of the parameters of analysis of the EEG such as frequency, amplitude, locus and interhemispheric coherence (symmetry and synchrony). As computer technology developed and faster computers and color monitors were available, the processing and display of analyzed EEG progressed until brain mapping was created.

There are a number of investigators who have contributed to the development of quantitative EEG. Some of the pioneers in this area are: Brazier (1961), John, Prichep, Fridman, and Easton (1988), Nuwer (1988a, 1988b), Gevins, Martin, Brickett, Desmond and Reuter (1994), Dumermuth and Molinari (1987), Duffy, Burchfiel, and Lombroso (1979), and Thatcher, Walker, and Guidice (1987), just to mention a few.

At present, no one questions the fact that the cerebral cortex is the site of mental functions (e.g., Penfield, 1954). The EEG is the method that records the function of this "enchanted loom." To paraphrase Sir Charles Sherrington, "The human brain is an enchanted loom where millions of flashing shuttles weave a dissolving pattern, always a meaningful pattern, though never an abiding one. It is as if the Milky Way entered upon some cosmic dance." EEG represents a window through which we can examine the functioning of this "machinery of the mind."

With the passage of time, EEG has shown its utility in the diagnosis and characterization of different pathologies that affect brain functioning with a well-defined application in neurology and an increasingly important one in neuropsychiatry.

Clinical neurophysiology evolved as a branch of medicine, and has become a specialty in itself. At present clinical neurophysiologists are grouped in local societies, which are part of the International Federation of Clinical Neurophysiology. There are also local councils that certify and support rational and careful use and application of this technique.

QUANTITATIVE EEG AND BRAIN MAPPING

The earliest researcher to anticipate the use of numerical computation in EEG was, not surprisingly, Hans Berger. Berger collaborated with a physicist, G. Dietsch, at the Institute of Technology and Physics in Jena, Germany. Together they worked on the theoretical basis for calculating the frequency spectrum of the EEG using the Fourier Transform. Although the theoretical basis was established by Berger and others, quantitative analysis of EEG had to wait until computers were available.

Grass and Gibbs (1938) and Bickford et al. (1973) were among the investigators who pioneered the area of computerized EEG. Dr. John Knott built a frequency analyzer in 1949 at the University of Iowa in collaboration with Drs. Henry, Gibbs and Grass. This group was the first to coin the term "CSA" for "continuous or compressed spectral array." Reginald Bickford at the University of California, San Diego (UCSD), developed and introduced the technique in 1972.

SPECTRAL ANALYSIS

One of the main features of EEG analysis corresponds to frequency. Traditionally, EEG frequency has been separated into frequency bands. These are:

Delta from 0.1 to 4 Hz

Theta from 4 to 8 Hz

Alpha from 8 to 13 Hz

Beta from 13 Hz up

Arranging EEG frequencies into bands was useful at the beginning of EEG analysis because of the limitations in visual analysis. Quantifying frequency by visual analysis is an almost impossible task. What we see in an EEG tracing is the result of a combination of frequencies, and visually quantifying a frequency would involve counting each component of a rhythm in one-second intervals. It would be very time consuming if not impossible to count every rhythm in an 8- or 16-channel tracing for the entire EEG record.

Fortunately, with computer analysis we are now able to quantify frequency very efficiently. Spectral decomposition of the EEG can be performed by Fourier analysis (Figure 1) which allows separation of various rhythms and estimation of their frequencies independently of each

FIGURE 1. The frequency spectrum can be obtained by performing Fourier analysis on a sample of raw EEG.

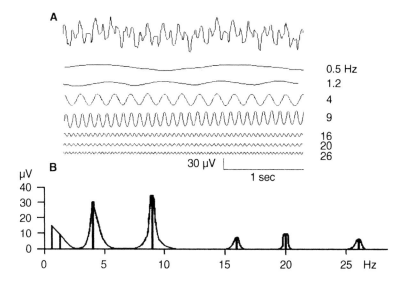

other, a task difficult to perform visually if several rhythmic activities occur simultaneously. Spectral analysis can also quantify the amount of activity in a frequency band.

Spectral analysis is based on the Fourier theorem, developed by a French mathematician in the 19th century who was obsessed with the idea of analyzing the propagation of heat through solids. In his treatise, *Théorie analytique de la chaleur (The Analytical Theory of Heat)*, Fourier (1822) employed trigonometric series, usually called the Fourier series, by means of which discontinuous functions can be expressed as the sum of an infinite series of sines and cosines.

In order to understand what Fourier analysis does to EEG, we could compare it to what happens to light when it passes through a glass prism. The beam of light decomposes into its main components thus obtaining the spectrum. Since the EEG is composed of a mixture of frequencies, its spectrum can also be obtained when processed by Fourier analysis.

Spectral analysis is only one of a wide variety of EEG analysis techniques, which includes analysis in the time and frequency domain. Power spectrum, coefficient of variation, coherence, ratios, period amplitude, and zero-crossing analysis are other analytic tools available, just to mention a few. There are more than ten thousand pages in the literature that cannot be summarized here. The interested reader is encouraged to consult Bickford et al. (1973), Brazier (1961), Dietsch (1932), Duffy (1986), Frost (1987), Gevins (1984), Hjorth (1986), John (1977), Kellaway and Petersen (1973), Nuwer and Jordan (1987), and Lopez da Silva et al. (1977).

BRAIN MAPPING

After digitizing and processing the EEG, there are also a number of display formats, which include colored bar displays, compressed spectral array, histograms, numerical tables, and topographic maps. Continuous or compressed spectral array (CSA) and brain mapping are the two most frequently used types of display for neurofeedback; therefore, we will focus on those.

CSA, developed by Reginald Bickford, consists of performing the spectral analysis of EEG, sorting the mixed frequencies into an orderly sequence from low to high (0.25 to 16 or more Hz) and plotting the graphs in a series, stacking one graph upon another in sequential temporal order (each epoch in chronological sequence).

Brain mapping involves the construction of a topographic map from the results of a multi-channel recording analysis. Interpolation is required to build these maps. It starts with the values measured at each electrode, then the values at intermediate locations are mathematically calculated by assuming smooth changes of the values between electrodes. Interpolated values can be displayed in different ways. Currently the most popular method assigns a color to a value, most commonly using a color spectrum scale, arranging the hues in an orderly fashion. Because phase is lost by performing frequency analysis through the use of Fourier analysis, the blue hues represent low values and the red hues high values (see Figure 2). When both positive and negative values are present as in voltage distribution maps, blue hues represent positive polarity and red hues negative polarity. (Note: In neurophysiology, negative is upward deflection of the trace, and positive is downward. See Figure 3.)

Brain maps can represent different types of analysis or information (i.e., voltage distribution at one instant of time, frequency data at one

FIGURE 2. Topographic maps in the frequency domain, arranged in frequency bands.

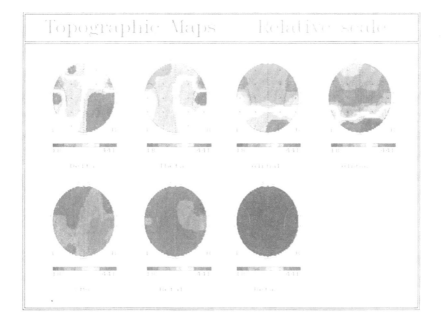

FIGURE 3. A transient event such as an epileptic spike can be precisely located by displaying a potential field distribution map in the time domain.

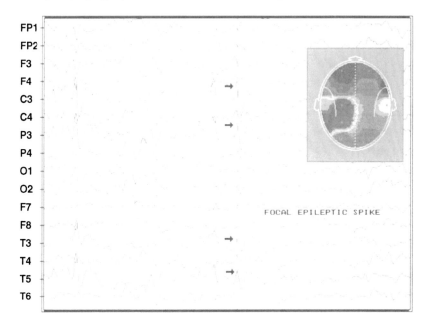

frequency or frequency bands, or a z-score of such time or frequency activity). Other more complex representations are also possible (Nuwer, 1988a, 1988b).

In the time domain, a map can be displayed at one instant of time, which is useful to analyze the potential field distribution of a phasic or transient event such as an epileptic spike. A series of maps can be displayed in progressive periods of time in order to assess how such events evolve over milliseconds of time (see Figure 4).

NORMATIVE DATABASES

The use of normative databases has become a common practice in the field of neurofeedback. Some of its advantages and limitations are discussed.

The use of normative databases is very important to the clinical neurophysiologist in terms of the information they provide in relation to quantification of different features of the EEG in normal populations,

FIGURE 4. By displaying a series of maps in progressive periods of time, propagation of a transient event along the cortex can be clearly assessed.

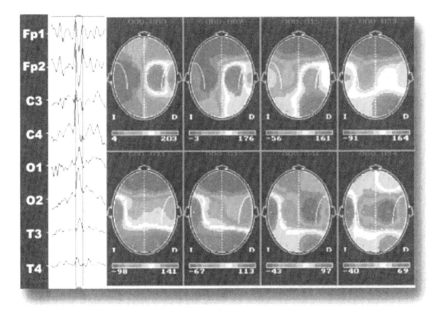

and also because they permit comparisons between populations of different pathologies. However, the assessment of the state of normality of an individual patient has a substantial array of difficulties.

The first difficulty relates to the technical quality of the data. It is of the utmost importance to have artifact-free samples of EEG. As Thatcher et al. (1987) pointed out, "The importance of this aspect of EEG data acquisition cannot be overstated." Even the small amount of artifacts easily tolerated in traditional EEG readings can wreak havoc in computer EEG analysis. It is a matter of "garbage in-garbage out" (Nuwer, 1988b).

Patients cannot always be compared to a normal database, even if the technical quality of a record is perfect. The normal subjects included in the databases may vary from the patient's own group in a number of ways that may affect results. Some databases have been collected on subjects rigorously excluding anyone who uses drugs or medicines, who has a history of any significant medical problem or head trauma, or who fails a physical examination. The population from which they are derived can influence databases.

It has been customary to use the normalcy criteria of Matousek and Petersen (1973) for membership in a normative QEEG database. This standard has been followed in the development of subsequent quantitative EEG databases by most authors. If one critically analyzes the required criteria for entry into the normative database (uneventful prenatal, perinatal and postnatal period, no disorders of consciousness, no head injury with cerebral symptoms, no history of central nervous diseases, no convulsions of emotion, febrile, or other nature, no abnormal deviation with regard to mental and physical development), then it is not difficult to see that this is an arbitrary standard for normalcy. To be strictly reliable and consistent, the "patients" compared to this reference normative database should also match the same criteria.

One may also question the clinical significance of a quantitative EEG feature lying outside normal limits. Even when data is collected in a technically adequate manner and a reasonably appropriate database is employed, an abnormality determined solely by statistics may not reflect a clinically meaningful abnormality. Electroencephalographers have long known about clinically meaningless normal variants in EEG records. These normal variants serve as reminders that EEG features may be statistically unusual in a group of normal subjects and may still be clinically meaningless. When quantitative EEG techniques rely on statistics and normal databases, they are predisposed to confusion between statistical and clinical abnormalities.

There are also further serious statistical issues that must be addressed. The types of statistics used in a simple z-score analysis are predisposed toward over-emphasizing some statistical abnormalities. The roots of this problem lie in part with statistical issues such as nongaussian distribution, the redundancy of testing similar data with separate tests, and a lack of independence of results from separate scalp sites. A simple z-score may show a result three standard deviations (SDs) above control values, and yet it does not necessarily imply that the patient's value lies outside the range of values observed in normal control subjects. Statistics can overemphasize abnormalities or erroneously find abnormality where none exists.

There are other important issues in EEG analysis that relate to the characterization of other parameters that are as important as frequency analysis. Some of them (waveform, regulation, manner of occurrence and reactivity) are better analyzed visually by an experienced clinical neurophysiologist. Also, even small amounts of artifact that can wreak havoc in computer EEG analysis provide important information in visual analysis for the clinical neurophysiologist in relation to the cooperation of the patient, the technical quality of the recording, the state of the patient, etc.

Relying only on databases to analyze an EEG, as has been previously discussed, has many disadvantages. Analysis and interpretation of the EEG is both a science and an art. On one hand, it is a rational and systematic process involving a series of orderly steps to characterize the electrical activity of the brain in terms of specific parameters such as frequency, amplitude, locus, interhemispheric coherence (symmetry and synchrony), waveform, regulation, manner of occurrence, and reactivity. On the other hand, the clinical neurophysiologist has to evaluate and correlate all these results in the light of a specific patient and conditions in order to derive a "clinical impression"; that is, an assessment of the probable significance of the EEG findings in relation to the patient's history and the clinical findings.

EEG analysis is so complicated that it requires arduous and constant training. A clinical neurophysiologist has to know what a normal EEG looks like at different ages (databases are useful for this), at different states and conditions, how all the different pathologies are expressed in the EEG, the normal variants, and the artifacts. If the clinical neurophysiologist wants to include quantitative EEG techniques, the reader needs to be expert as well in computer analysis of EEG. The interpretation of EEG requires substantial clinical experience. The interpreter must understand also that the increased power of these techniques also increases their potential for misinterpretation.

SPECIFIC TRAINING PROTOCOLS FOR NEUROTHERAPY

Specific training protocols for different disorders or symptoms have been widely used since the beginning of neurotherapy practice. Sterman (1982) found that training SMR in epileptic cats was useful in lowering seizure frequency. Lubar (1997) found that children with ADD benefited with SMR training. Since then, many practitioners have come up with different protocols, most of them arbitrary and discovered by chance, and without clear and scientific foundation. These types of findings, although they have provided important information and have proven to be useful in different pathologies, have caused conceptual errors in interpretation. There is a tendency to oversimplify brain function and to interpret it in a reductionist way by pretending to explain it in a direct cause-effect way. Practitioners tend to relate alpha with relaxation, SMR with attention, and specific frequencies with specific brain functions. In brain neurophysiology this is not the case. As one can see in electroencephalography, there is no relationship between a specific frequency and a specific disease or symptom. As we have learned from qEEG, a brain frequency such as alpha or beta is actually a mixture of frequencies; millions of cortical generators are contributing to a specific frequency. We now know with certainty that there is a correlation between cortical topography and brain functions and not one with specific brain frequencies. Neurophysiology has provided important information in this respect.

Some neurofeedback practitioners have even tried to further oversimplify neurotherapy by trying to obtain a description of symptoms and decide by the application of an initial interview and a series of clinical questions if the brain is in a specific brain state or in a specific state of performance so they train frequencies to acquire a "high performance" brain state. That is an even more inexact approach. One could easily reach wrong conclusions such as thinking that a patient with migraine is in a brain state dominated by fast brainwaves. Clinical neurophysiologists have shown that migraine patients actually have slow waves in their EEGs.

The brain is a very complex organ, with a complexity that we cannot even conceive with our imagination. Knowledge about the brain has increased tremendously in the last two decades. Technical development has provided more precise and powerful tools to the fields of neurophysiology, neuropharmacology, neuropsychology, and other neurodisciplines to understand the most complex organ known in nature. Recently, we have seen an ever increasing dialogue between disciplines. We see more neurologists interested in psychological processes and more psychologists looking for an "organic" basis for the patient's complaints. At the end, there is no division. Brain and behavior are part of the same whole. This organ is so complex that there is no single individual who can cover all aspects of knowledge. We have to dedicate a whole human life just to understand the tip of the iceberg of only one point of view. That is why we specialize in a specific field of knowledge so we become psychophysiologists, neuropharmacologists, neurophysiologists, etc.

Neurofeedback is a very special discipline because it stands right at the landmark of brain and behavior so it deals with all the complexities of brain function and brain functions.

A PROPOSAL FOR A "CLINICAL APPROACH TO NEUROTHERAPY"

We have discussed some important aspects in relation to a substantial array of difficulties that the use of databases has in order to assess the state of normality of an individual patient. We have also mentioned the weakness of the conceptual foundation and the arbitrary approach of the use of specific protocols in neurotherapy. Both approaches share the intention to simplify what is not simplifiable–that is understanding and manipulating brain function. On one hand, data bases by the use of statistics pretend to show anatomical locations that are most deviant from normal when compared to a group of "normal" individuals, in an effort to individualize neurotherapy treatment. One frequent question that arises between neurofeedback practitioners who use this approach is whether one should train an area that is statistically deviant from the norm although it does not correlate with the symptoms of the patient. In this case, who is right, the statistics or the patient?

If the investigator relies upon inferential statistics in an isolated way without verifying the clinical meaning, a fundamental error of clinical interpretation can occur. Often investigators do not question the clinical meaning of the inferential statistics because numbers are supposed to be exact and true in nature.

If neurofeedback is going to be used in patient care, the model of therapeutic neurofeedback that should be used is what I call a *clinical approach* to neurofeedback. This means collecting and analyzing an EEG in a conventional and quantitative way using a trained professional, then evaluating and correlating all the results of a specific patient and specific conditions to derive a "clinical impression" in concert with a good clinical history, physical exam, and psychological or neuropsychological tests. That is, a neurofeedback protocol should be based upon an assessment of the probable significance of the EEG findings in relation to the patient's history and clinical findings. Building an individualized neurofeedback training protocol should take into account the relevant EEG findings, including the training of specific frequencies which have been clearly demonstrated to improve different states and symptoms, such as inattention or epilepsy (Lubar, 1997; Sterman, 1982).

This proposed approach is a very complex one, but not as complex as the brain. It requires a multidisciplinary team of professionals, not only to build a neurofeedback training protocol, but to make a correct medical and psychological diagnosis and to treat a patient in a multidisciplinary way, not forgetting that neurofeedback is just another piece of the therapeutic procedure, as is psychotherapy, pharmacotherapy, etc.

AN ETHICAL ISSUE

There is significant evidence for a neurological effect of neuro-feedback. Abrams and Kandel (1988) found that there is activity-dependent enhancement of pre-synaptic facilitation in classical conditioning. They found that action potentials allow calcium (Ca^{++}) to move into sensory neurons. This influx of Ca^{++} acting through calmodulin is thought to amplify the activation of adenyl cyclase by serotonin and other modulatory transmitters thus producing greater amounts of transmitter release.

Another piece of evidence comes from the work of Merzenich et al. (1983) who demonstrated that the brain cortex architecture can be modified by the manipulation of external stimuli. Cortical maps are subject to constant modification on the basis of environmental influence.

Jenkins et al. (1990) demonstrated reorganization of the cortex through learning activities. They encouraged monkeys to use their middle three fingers at the expense of other fingers by having them obtain food by contacting a rotating disc with only the middle fingers. After several thousand disc rotations, the area in the cortex devoted to the middle three fingers was greatly expanded. Now, there is abundant evidence that learning produces structural changes in the cortex.

Previous evidence strongly suggests that neurofeedback can be an important tool for neuroplasticity. As has been clearly demonstrated, (e.g., Goldensohn, 1979) EEG activity is generated in the pyramidal cells of the cortex. As pointed out previously, there is evidence of synaptic facilitation and structural modification of the cerebral cortex by external stimulation and learning, so it is most probable that the changes obtained in EEG activity with neurofeedback reflect structural changes in the cell generators.

As pointed out at the beginning of this paper, neurofeedback provides an opportunity for the integration of neurological and psychological sciences. Neurofeedback lies right at the interface of mind and brain interaction. It seems to integrate the psychological aspect of healing, the positive attitude, and the neurological aspect that relates to neuro-plasticity.

If neurofeedback can bring about structural modification of the brain–as growing evidence suggests–then an ethical issue has to be outlined. So far, there have been no reports of iatrogenesis (a harmful effect produced by the healer or the healing process) through the use of neurofeedback. However, this does not guarantee that there cannot be harmful effects through changing the physiology and probably the structure of a brain area where such changes are not needed.

Homeostasis is a fundamental natural system preserving health. If neurofeedback can change homeostatic processes, then it is of the utmost importance to maintain a very careful and responsible attitude in order to help nature and not to disrupt it.

REFERENCES

Abrams, T. W., & Kandel, E. (1988). Is contiguity detection in classical conditioning a system or a cellular property? Learning in Aplysia suggests a possible molecular site. *Trends in Neuroscience, 11*, 128-135.

Berger, H. (1969). On the electroencephalogram of man (translated by P. Gloor). *Electroencephalography and Clinical Neurophysiology, 28* (Suppl.), 267-287.

Brazier, M. A. B. (1961). Computer techniques in EEG analysis. *Electroencephalography and Clinical Neurophysiology, 20* (Suppl.), 2-6.

Bickford, R. G., Brimm, J., Berger, L., & Aung, M. (1973). Applications of compressed spectral array in clinical EEG. In P. Kellaway & I. Petersen (Eds.), *Automation of clinical electroencephalography* (pp. 55-64). New York: Raven Press.

Dietsch, G. (1932). Fourier-Analyse von Elektrenkephalogrammen des Menschen. Pflugers Archive. *European Journal of Physiology, 230*, 106-112.

Duffy, F. H. (1986). *Topographic mapping of brain electrical activity.* Boston: Butterworths.

Duffy, F. H., Burchfiel, J. L., & Lombroso, C. T. (1979). Brain electrical activity mapping (BEAM): A method for extending the clinical utility of EEG and evoked potential data. *Annals of Neurology, 5*, 309-321.

Dumermuth, G., & Molinari, L. (1987). Spectral analysis of EEG background activity. In A. S. Gevins & A. Remond (Eds.), *Handbook of electroencephalography and clinical neurophysiology: Vol. 1. Methods of analysis of brain electrical and magnetic signals* (pp. 85-130). Amsterdam: Elsevier.

Eccles, J. C. (1951). Interpretation of action potentials evoked in the cerebral cortex. *Electroencephalography and Clinical Neurophysiology, 3*, 449-464.

Fourier, J. (1822). *Théorie analytique de la chaleur.* A. Paris. ISBN: 2-87647-046-2.

Frost, J. D., Jr. (1987). Mimetic techniques. In: A. S. Gevins & A. Remond (Eds.), *Handbook of electroencephalography and clinical neurophysiology: Vol. 1. Methods of analysis of brain electrical and magnetic signals* (pp. 195-209). Amsterdam: Elsevier.

Gevins, A., Martin, N., Brickett, P., Desmond, J., & Reuter, B. (1994). High resolution EEG: 124 channel recording spatial deblurring and MRI integration. *Electroencephalography and Clinical Neurophysiology, 90*, 337-358.

Gevins, A. S. (1984). Analysis of the electromagnetic signals of the human brain: Milestones, obstacles, and goals. *IEEE Transactions on Biomedical Engineering, 31,* 833-850.

Gloor, P. (1969). *Hans Berger on the electroencephalogram of man.* Amsterdam: Elsevier.

Goldensohn, E. S. (1979). Neurophysiologic substrates of EEG activity. In D. Klass & D. Daly (Eds.), *Current practice of clinical electroencephalography* (pp. 421-440). New York: Raven Press.

Grass. A. M., & Gibbs, F. A. (1938). A Fourier transform of the electroencephalogram. *Journal of Neurophysiology, 1,* 521-526.

Hjorth, B. (1986). Physical aspects of EEG data as a basis for topographic mapping. In F. H. Duffy (Ed.), *Topographic mapping of brain electrical activity* (pp. 175-193). Boston: Butterworths.

Jenkins, W. M., Merzenich, M. M., Ochs, M. T., Allard, T., & Guic-Robles, E. (1990). Functional reorganization of primary somatosensory cortex in adult owl monkeys after behaviorally controlled tactile stimulation. *Journal of Neurophysiology, 63,* 82-104.

John E. R., Prichep, L. S., Fridman, J., & Easton, P. (1988). Neurometrics: Computer-assisted differential diagnosis of brain dysfunctions. *Science, 239,* 162-169.

John, E. R. (1977). *Neurometrics: Clinical applications of quantitative electrophysiology.* New York: Wiley.

Kamiya, J. (1968). Conscious control of brain waves. *Psychology Today, 1,* 56-60.

Kellaway, P., & Petersén, I. (Eds.). (1973). *Automation of clinical electroencephalography.* New York: Raven Press.

Lopes da Silva, F. H., van Hulten, K., Lommen, J. G., van Leeuwen, W. S., van Veelen, C. W. M. et al. (1977). Automatic detection and localization of epileptic foci. *Electroencephalography and Clinical Neurophysiology, 43,* 1-13.

Lubar, J. F. (1991). Discourse on the development of EEG diagnostics and biofeedback treatment for attention-deficit/hyperactivity disorders. *Biofeedback and Self-Regulation, 16,* 201-225.

Lubar, J. F. (1997). Neocortical dynamics: Implications for understanding the role of neurofeedback and related techniques for the enhancement of attention. *Applied Psychophysiology and Biofeedback, 22,* 111-126.

Matousek, M., & Petersen, I. (1973). Frequency analysis of the EEG in normal children and adolescents. In P. Kellaway & I. Petersen (Eds.), *Automation of clinical electroencephalography* (p. 75). New York: Raven Press.

Merzenich, M. M., Kass, J. H., Wall, J., Nelson, R. J., Sur, M., & Felleman, D. (1983). Topographic reorganization of somatosensory cortical areas 3B and 1 in adult monkeys following restricted deafferentation. *Neuroscience, 8,* 33-55.

Nuwer, M. R., & Jordan, S. E. (1987). The centrifugal effect and other spatial artifacts of topographic EEG mapping. *Journal of Clinical Neurophysiology, 4,* 321-326.

Nuwer, M. R. (1988a). Quantitative EEG: I. Techniques and problems of frequency analysis and topographic mapping. *Journal of Clinical Neurophysiology, 5,* 1-43.

Nuwer, M. R. (1988b). Quantitative EEG: II. Frequency analysis and topographic mapping in clinical settings. *Journal of Clinical Neurophysiology, 5,* 45-86.

Ochs, L. (1992). EEG treatment of addictions. *Biofeedback, 20* (1), 8-16.

Oken, B. S., & Chiappa, K. H. (1986). Statistical issues concerning computerized analysis of brainwave topography. *Annals of Neurology, 19*, 493-494.

Penfield, W., & Herbert, J. (1954). *Epilepsy and the functional anatomy of the human brain.* Boston: Little, Brown.

Peniston, E. G., & Kulkosky, P. J. (1989). Alpha-theta brainwave training and endorphin levels of alcoholics. *Alcoholism: Clinical and Experimental Research, 13* (2), 271-279.

Romano-Micha, J. (2000). Reflections about brain mapping and neurofeedback: A perspective from Mexico. *Biofeedback, 28* (2), 11-13.

Rosenfeld, J. P. (1992). "EEG" treatment of addictions: Commentary on Ochs, Peniston, and Kulkosky. *Biofeedback, 20* (2), 12-17.

Rosenfeld, J. P. (1997). EEG biofeedback of frontal alpha asymmetry in affective disorders. *Biofeedback, 25* (1), 8-25.

Rozelle, R., & Budzynski, T. H. (1995). Neurotherapy for stroke rehabilitation: A single case study. *Biofeedback and Self-Regulation, 20*, 211-228.

Sterman, M. B., & Friar, L. (1972). Suppression of seizures in epileptic following sensorimotor EEG feedback training. *Electroencephalography and Clinical Neurophysiology, 33*, 89-95.

Thatcher, R. W., Walker, R. A., & Guidice, S. (1987). Human cerebral hemispheres develop at different rates and ages. *Science, 236*, 1110-1113.

Walter, D. O. (1963). Spectral analysis for electroencephalograms: Mathematical determination of neurophysiological relationships from records of limited duration. *Experimental Neurology, 8*, 155-181.

Quantitative EEG Normative Databases: Validation and Clinical Correlation

Robert W. Thatcher, PhD
Rebecca A. Walker, BS
Carl J. Biver, PhD
Duane N. North, MS
Richard Curtin, MA

SUMMARY. The quantitative digital electroencephalogram (QEEG) was recorded from 19 scalp locations from 625 screened and evaluated normal individuals ranging in age from two months to 82 years. After editing to remove artifact, one-year to five-year groupings were selected to produce different average age groups. Estimates of gaussian distributions and logarithmic transforms of the digital EEG were used to establish approximate gaussian distributions when necessary for different

Robert W. Thatcher is affiliated with the NeuroImaging Laboratory, Bay Pines VA Medical Center and the Department of Neurology, University of South Florida College of Medicine, Tampa, FL.

Rebecca A. Walker, Carl J. Biver, Duane N. North and Richard Curtin are affiliated with the NeuroImaging Laboratory, Bay Pines VA Medical Center.

Address correspondence to: Robert W. Thatcher, NeuroImaging Lab, VA Medical Center, Building 23, Room 117, Bay Pines, FL 33744 (E-mail: robert@appliedneuroscience.com).

The authors want to acknowledge the assistance and feedback of Lukasz Knopka, Joel Lubar, Grant Bright and D. Corydon Hammond for their independent evaluations of the normative databases.

variables and age groupings. The sensitivity of the lifespan database was determined by gaussian cross-validation for any selection of age range in which the average percentage of Z-scores ± 2 standard deviations (SD) equals approximately 2.3% and the average percentage for ± 3 SD equals approximately 0.13%. It was hypothesized that measures of gaussian cross-validation of Z-scores is a common metric by which the statistical sensitivity of any normative database for any age grouping can be calculated. This theory was tested by computing eyes-closed and eyes-open average reference and current source density norms and independently cross-validating and comparing to the linked ears norms. The results indicate that age-dependent digital EEG normative databases are reliable and stable and behave like different gaussian lenses that spatially focus the electroencephalogram. Clinical correlations of a normative database are determined by content validation and correlation with neuropsychological test scores and discriminate accuracy. Non-parametric statistics were presented as an important aid to establish the alpha level necessary to reject a hypothesis and to estimate Type I and Type II errors, especially when there are multiple comparisons of an individual's EEG to any normative EEG database. *[Article copies available for a fee from The Haworth Document Delivery Service: 1-800-HAWORTH. E-mail address: <docdelivery@haworthpress.com> Website: <http://www.HaworthPress.com> © 2003 by The Haworth Press, Inc. All rights reserved.]*

KEYWORDS. EEG normative databases, gaussian distributions, error estimates

INTRODUCTION

There are many potential uses of a normative electroencephalogram (EEG) database. Among the most important it is a statistical "guess" as to the "error rate" or to the probability of finding a particular patient's EEG measure within a reference normal population. Most other uses of a reference EEG database also involve statistics and the same statistics that all of modern clinical medicine relies upon. For example, null hypothesis testing, measures of reliability, sensitivity, power, predictive validity, content validity, etc., all depend on specific assumptions and statistical procedures.

Predictive accuracy and error rates depend on the data that make up a given EEG database and the statistics of the database. The statistical foundations of the scientific method were visited by the Supreme Court in Daubert (1993) regarding admissibility of scientific evidence. The four *Daubert* factors for scientific standards of admissibility in Federal

Courts are: (a) hypothesis testing, (b) error estimates of reliability and validity, (c) peer-reviewed publications and (d) general acceptance (Mahle, 2001; Thatcher, Biver, & North, 2003. These four *Daubert* factors have already been met for several EEG normative databases (John, Prichep, & Easton, 1987; Duffy, Hughes, Miranda, Bernad, & Cook, 1994; Thatcher, Walker, & Guidice, 1987; Thatcher et al., 2003). The minimal standards of publication are: (a) inclusion/exclusion criteria, (b) methods to remove artifact and adequate sample sizes per age groups, (c) demographically representative (e.g., balanced gender, ethnicity, socioeconomic status, etc.), (d) means and standard deviations as being normally distributed or gaussian including gaussian cross-validation, and (e) content validity by correlations with clinical measures, neuropsychological test scores and school achievement scores, etc., as validation. Predictive validity is determined by regression and classification statistics. Predictive validity relates to the estimation of classification accuracy, clinical severity, clinical outcome, etc. The sensitivity and specificity of any EEG database is directly proportional to its adherence to the established statistical principals in the history of statistics (Hayes, 1973).

The purpose of this paper is to review the current NeuroGuide normative database which uses the University of Maryland EEG normative database in which the methods and clinical validity have been published (Thatcher, McAlaster, Lester, Horst, & Cantor, 1983; Thatcher, Walker, & Guidice, 1987; Thatcher, 1991, 1992, 1994, 1998) and then to illustrate step by step the procedures that NeuroGuide used to meet measurable standards of reliability and validity of clinical correlation using the University of Maryland EEG data as an example of how to construct a normative database. Similar steps to construct a normative EEG database were described for the NYU School of Medicine database by John, Prichep, and Easton (1987). However, important differences in tests of clinical validity and age groupings were used in comparison to the NeuroGuide methods described in this paper. The reader is encouraged to read the John et al. (1987) paper in order to broaden understanding about the foundations of EEG normative databases.

GENERAL METHOD
TO PRODUCE A VALID NORMATIVE EEG DATABASE

Figure 1 is an illustration of a step-by-step procedure by which any normative EEG database can be validated and sensitivities calculated.

FIGURE 1. Illustration of the step by step procedure to gaussian cross-validate and then validate by correlations with clinical measures in order to estimate the predictive and content validity of any EEG normative database. The feedback connections between gaussian cross validation and the means and standard deviations refers to transforms to approximate gaussian if the non-transformed data is less gaussian. The clinical correlation and validation arrow to the montage stage represents repetition of clinical validation to a different montage or reference or condition such as eyes-open, active tasks, eyes-closed, etc., to the adjustments and understanding of the experimental design(s).

Normative Database Validation Steps

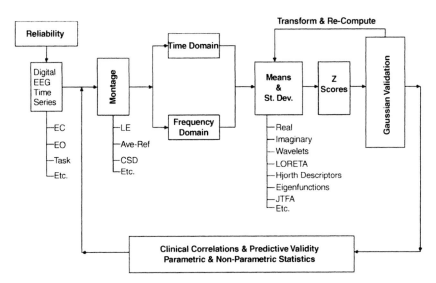

The left side of the figure is the edited and artifact clean and reliable digital EEG time series which may be re-referenced or re-montaged, which is then analyzed in either the time domain or the frequency domain.

The selected normal subjects are grouped by age with a sufficiently large sample size. The means and standard deviations of the EEG time series and/or frequency domain analyses are computed for each age group. Transforms are applied to approximate a gaussian distribution of the EEG measures that comprise the means. Once approximation to gaussian is completed, Z-scores are computed for each subject in the database and leave one out gaussian cross-validation is computed in order to arrive at optimum gaussian cross-validation sensitivity. Finally the gaussian validated norms are subjected to content and predictive validation procedures such as correlation with neuropsychological test scores and intelligence, etc., and also discriminant analyses and neural networks and outcome statistics, etc. The content validations are with respect to clinical measures such as intelligence, neuropsychological test scores, school achievement, clinical outcomes, etc. The predictive validations are with respect to the discriminative, statistical or neural network clinical classification accuracy. Both parametric and non-parametric statistics are used to determine the content and predictive validity of a normative EEG database.

STEPS TO PRODUCE A NORMATIVE EEG DATABASE

The steps in Figure 1 can be repeated for different selections of subjects, different selections of derived measures and different frequency and spatio-temporal transforms for any normative QEEG database. The gaussian distribution is emphasized because most other distributions, such as the chi square distribution, F distribution, t distribution and Kamma distribution can be mathematically transformed into a gaussian distribution (Hayes, 1973). Also, the scientific standards of parametric statistics are best applied when means and standard deviations are gaussian distributed (John et al., 1987; John, Prichep, Fridman, & Easton, 1988; Duffy et al., 1994; Thatcher, 1998; Thatcher, Biver & North, 2003).

SUBJECT AND VARIABLE SELECTION

Nineteen (19) channels of EEG and an Electro-Oculogram (EOG) channel, a two-hour battery of evoked potential tests and active challenges, psychometric tests, dietary evaluations, anthrometric measurements, demographic and trace element measurements from a population of 1,015 rural and urban children were collected (Thatcher et al., 1983; Thatcher et al., 1987; Thatcher, 1998). The principal goal of this project was to evaluate the effects of environmental toxins on child development and to determine the extent to which good or poor diets may ameliorate or exacerbate the deleterious effects of environmental toxins. Two data acquisition centers were established, one at the rural University of Maryland Eastern Shore campus and one at the urban campus of the University of Maryland School of Medicine in Baltimore, Maryland. Identical data acquisition systems were built and calibrated; a staff was trained using uniform procedures and clinical and psychometric protocols were utilized in the recruitment of normal subjects. A total of 1,015 subjects ranging in age from two months to 82 years were tested during the period from 1979 to 1987. Of these subjects, 564 met the criteria of normalcy and were included in the normative reference database (Thatcher et al., 1987; Thatcher, 1998). In 2000 the original digital EEG was revisited and a different selection of individuals was selected that also spanned the same interval from two months to 82 years and included 61 additional adult subjects to increase the total sample size to 625 subjects. The expanded selection contained more individuals between the ages of 25 and 55 years of age.

Figure 2 shows the number of subjects per year in the normative EEG lifespan database. It can be seen that the largest number of subjects are in the younger ages (e.g., 1 to 14 years, N = 470) when the EEG is changing most rapidly. As mentioned previously, a proportionately smaller number of subjects represent the adult age range from 14 to 83 years (N = 155). Fifteen one-year groupings of subjects were computed with reasonable sample sizes from birth to 15 years of age. Thirteen out of the 15 one-year age groups have N > 20 with the largest sample size at age 3 to 4 years (N = 45). The smallest one-year sample size was between age 2 and 3 (N = 16).

For each subject, original selections of the digital EEG occurred by different artifact procedures involving the use of NeuroGuide editing selections (www.appliedneuroscience.com). Original arrangements of coherence, phase, amplitude asymmetry and relative power also occurred when comparing the database to previous publications (Thatcher et al., 1987; Thatcher, 1998). Although different selections of digital EEG values and different arrangements of the original digital EEG have occurred since 1987, the gaussian validations and sensitivities of the previous databases and the current 2003 database are all similar and equally valid and gaussian distributed within a 90 to 99 percent range depending on the measure. The original digital EEG, the subjects and neuropsychological test scores that were measured from 1979 to 1987 are the same.

INCLUSION/EXCLUSION CRITERIA, DEMOGRAPHICS AND GENDER

Details of the neuropsychological testing, demographic and sampling of the normative 1987 EEG database were previously published in

FIGURE 2. The number of subjects per year in the Lifespan EEG reference normative database. The database is a "life-span" database with two months of age being the youngest subject and 82.3 years of age being the oldest subject. This figure shows the number of subjects constituting mean values which range from a mean of 0.5 years to 62.6 years of age and constituting a total of 625 subjects.

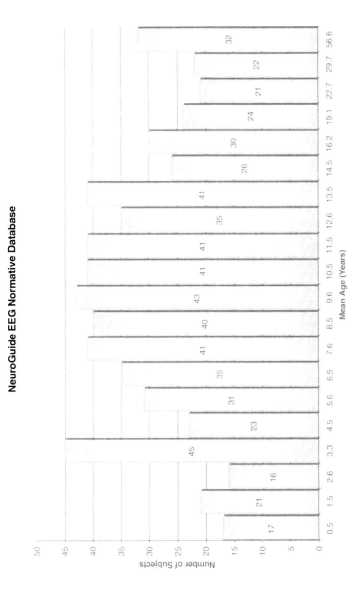

NeuroGuide EEG Normative Database

Thatcher et al. (1983), Thatcher and Krause (1986), Thatcher et al. (1987) and Thatcher (1998). Some but not all of the 61 adults added in 2000 to 2001 were given neuropsychological tests and other evaluations to help determine "normalcy"; however, all of the subjects were interviewed and filled out a history and neurological questionnaire. All of the 61 added adults were gainfully employed as professors, graduate students, and other successfully employed adults without a history of neurological problems. Normalcy for the age range from two months to 18 years was determined by one or more exclusion/inclusion criteria: (a) a neurological history questionnaire given to the child's parents and/or filled out by each subject, (b) psychometric evaluation of IQ and/or school achievement, (c) for children the teacher and class room performance as determined by school grades and teacher reports and presence of environmental toxins such as lead or cadmium. A neurological questionnaire was obtained from all of the adult subjects more than 18 years of age and those in which information was available about a history of problems as an adult were excluded.

INTELLIGENCE AND SCHOOL ACHIEVEMENT CRITERIA

Psychometric, demographic and socioeconomic status measures were obtained from each child, adolescent and for some of the adults. Different psychometric tests were administered depending upon the age of the child. There is little reliability in the IQ tests of infants; however, when possible the infant's Apgar score was obtained and the Vineland Social Maturity Scale test was administered (age birth to 2 years, 4 months). From age 2 years to 3.99 years, the McCarthy Intelligence Scale Test was administered; from age 4.0 years to 5.99 years the Wechsler Pre-School and Primary Scale of Intelligence (WIPPSI) test was administered; from age 6.0 years to 16.99 years the Wechsler Intelligence Scale for Children (WISC-R, 1972) was administered and from age 17.0 years to adulthood the Wechsler Adult Intelligence Scale test (WAIS) was administered. In addition to intelligence tests, the Wide Range School Achievement test (WRAT) was administered to the school age children and grade cards were obtained from the public school systems. Finally, a variety of neuropsychological tests were administered including the pegboard test of skilled motor movements, the Stott, Moyes and Henderson Test of Motor Impairment (MIT) and a eight-item laterality test (see Thatcher, Lester, McAlaster, & Horst, 1982; Thatcher et al., 1983 for further details).

The criteria for entry into the normative database for those subjects given IQ tests and school achievement tests were:

1. A Full Scale IQ > 70.
2. WRAT School Achievement Scores > 89 on at least two subtests (i.e., reading, spelling, arithmetic) or demonstrated success in these subjects.
3. A grade point average of 'C' or better in the major academic classes (e.g., English, mathematics, science, social studies and history).

DEMOGRAPHIC CHARACTERISTICS

It is important that the demographic mixture of males and females, different ethnic groups and socioeconomic status be reasonably representative of expected North American clientele. The normative EEG database is made up of 58.9% males, 41.1% females, 71.4% whites, 24.2% blacks and 3.2% oriental. Socioeconomic status (SES) was measured by the Hollingshead four factor scale (see Thatcher et al., 1983 for details).

TIME OF DAY AND OTHER MISCELLANEOUS FACTORS

There are many uncontrollable factors that influence the frequency spectrum of the EEG. In general these factors are all confounded and it would require an enormously expensive and large sample size to control each factor individually. Even if one could control each factor, such experimental control would preclude the practical use of a database since each patient's EEG would have to be acquired in a precisely matching manner. Statistical randomization is one of the best methods to deal with these uncontrollable and miscellaneous factors. Statistical randomization of a database involves randomly varying time of day of EEG acquisition, time between food intake and EEG acquisition, food content and EEG acquisition, etc., across ages, sex and demographics. Because these factors are confounded with each other, randomization with a sufficient sample size will result in increased variance but, nonetheless, convergence toward a gaussian distribution. Such convergence, even in the face of increased variance, still allows quantitative comparisons to be made and false positive and false negative error rates (i.e., sensitivity) to be calculated. The method of statistical randomization of miscellaneous factors was used in the Matousek and Petersen (1973); Thatcher, Walker, Gerson, and Geisler (1989); John et al. (1988); and Duffy et al. (1994) EEG normative databases.

DIGITAL ELECTROENCEPHALOGRAPHIC
RECORDING PROCEDURES

EEG was recorded and digitized at a rate of 100 Hz from the 19 leads of the International 10/20 system of electrode placement referenced to linked ear lobes and one bipolar EOG lead (i.e., a total of 20 channels; Thatcher et al., 1983; Thatcher & Krause, 1986; Thatcher et al., 1987; Thatcher, 1998). When head size was amenable, the data were acquired using a stretchable electrode cap (Electrocap International, Inc.). When head sizes were either too small or too large for the electrocap, then the electrophysiological data were acquired by applying standard silver disk Grass electrodes. Amplifiers were calibrated using sine wave calibration signals and standardized procedures. A permanent record made before and after each test session. The frequency response of the amplifiers was approximately three decibels down at 0.5 Hz and 30 Hz. Impedance was measured and recorded for each electrode and efforts were made to obtain impedance measures less than 10 K ohms (most of the impedances were < 5 K ohms) for all subjects.

ARTIFACT REMOVAL
AND QUALITY CONTROL PROCEDURES

EEG recording lengths varied from 58.6 seconds to 40 minutes. Artifact rejection involved using the NeuroGuide editing procedures in which a one- to two-second template of "clean" or "artifact free" EEG was selected. This template was then used to compute matching amplitudes of EEG using flexible criteria of equal amplitudes to amplitudes that are 1.25 or 1.5 times larger in amplitude. The decision as to which clean EEG sample multiplier to use was determined by the length of the sample 58.6 seconds as a minimum, visual inspection of the digital EEG and when split-half reliability > 0.97. After multiple visual inspections and selection of "clean" EEG samples, the edited samples varied in length from 58.6 seconds to 142.4 seconds. Average split-half reliability = 0.982 for the selected EEG in the database. Care was taken to in-spect the EEG from each subject in order to eliminate drowsiness or other state changes in the EEG which may have been present in the longer EEG recording sessions. No evidence of sharp waves or epileptogenic events was present in any of the EEG records.

RE-MONTAGE TO THE SURFACE LAPLACIAN AND AVERAGE REFERENCE

The average reference involved summing the voltages across all 19 leads for each time point and dividing this value into the microvolt digital value from each lead at each time point. This procedure produced a digital EEG time series that was then submitted to the same age groupings and power spectral analyses and the same gaussian normative evaluations as for linked ears (see Figure 1).

The reference free surface Laplacian or current source density (CSD) was computed using the spherical harmonic Fourier expansion of the EEG scalp potentials to estimate the CSD directed at right angles to the surface of the scalp in the vicinity of each scalp location (Pascual-Marqui, Gonzalez-Andino, Valdes-Sosa, & Biscay-Lirio, 1988). The CSD is the second spatial derivative or Laplacian of the scalp electrical potentials which is independent of the linked ear reference itself. The Laplacian is reference free in that it is only dependent upon the electrical potential gradients surrounding each electrode. The Laplacian transform also produces a new digital EEG time series of estimates of current source density in microamperes that were also submitted to the same age groupings spectral analyses (see Figure 1).

COMPLEX DEMODULATION COMPUTATIONS

The mathematical details of both the FFT and complex demodulation are described in Otnes and Enochson (1972), Bendat and Piersol (1980), and Thatcher (1998). The NeuroGuide EEG norms use both the complex demodulation and the FFT so that users can compare and contrast both methods in the same subject or application. Complex demodulation is a time domain digital method of spectral analysis whereas the fast Fourier transform (FFT) is a frequency domain method. These two methods are related by the fact they both involve sines and cosines and both operate in the complex domain and in this way represent the same mathematical descriptions of the power spectrum. The advantage of complex demodulation is that it is a time domain method and less sensitive to artifact and it does not require even integers of the power of 2 as does the FFT. The FFT integrates frequency over the entire epoch length and requires windowing functions which can dramatically affect the power values whereas complex demodulation does not require windowing (Otnes & Enochson, 1972).

FFT LINKED EARS, AVERAGE REFERENCE AND LAPLACIAN

The 100 samples per second digital EEG were first cubic-spline interpolated to 128 samples per second using standard procedures (Press, Teukolsky, Vettering, & Flannery, 1994). The second step was to high pass filter the EEG at 40 Hz to eliminate any possible splice artifact that may have been produced by appending short segments of EEG using the NeuroGuide editor. The third step was to compute the FFT power spectral density. Two-second epochs were used to compute the FFT power spectral density thus producing 0.5 Hz resolution and a Cosine window was used for each FFT computation. The 25% sliding window method of Kaiser and Sterman (2001) was used to compute the FFT normative database for linked ears, average reference and Laplacian estimator of current source density (CSD) in which successive two-second epochs (i.e., 256 points) were overlapped by 500 millisecond steps (64 points) in order to minimize the effects of the FFT windowing procedure. The FFT power spectral density and the average of the two second overlapping epochs produced a total of 61 frequency values in $\mu v^2/Hz$ from 0 to 30 Hz at 0.5 Hz resolution.

This procedure was repeated for linked ears, average reference and Laplacian digital values for both the eyes-closed and eyes-open conditions, thus producing for a given subject a total of six different 61 point FFT power spectral density values. These values were then used to compute means and standard deviations for different age groups. The FFT normative database did not use sliding averages of age in the manner of the complex demodulation database (see Thatcher, 1998). Instead, five sequential age groupings were selected to cover the age range from two months to 82 years. The age groupings were: (a) two months to 5.99 years (N = 122), (b) 6.0 years to 9.99 years (N = 147), (c) 10 to 13 years (N = 72), (d) 13 to 16 years (N = 117) and (e) 16 to 82 years (N = 167).

AMPLIFIER AND DIGITAL MATCHING

The frequency characteristics of all amplifiers differ to some extent, especially in the < 3 Hz and > 20 Hz frequency range and there are no universal standards that all EEG amplifier manufacturers must abide by. Therefore, amplifier filter and gain characteristics must be equilibrated to the amplifier gains and frequency characteristics of the normative EEG amplifiers that acquired the EEG in the first place. A simple method to accomplish this is to inject into each amplifier system microvolt sine waves from 0 to 40 Hz in single Hz steps and at three different microvolt amplitudes. The ratio of the frequency response characteristics between the normative EEG amplifiers and the amplifier characteristics by which EEG was measured from a patient can be used as equilibration factors to approximately match the frequency characteristics of the norms.

It should be kept in mind that even with matching of amplifier characteristics within 3 to 5% error, the enormous variability in skull thickness effects the amplitude and frequency characteristics of the EEG itself far more than slight differences in amplifier characteristics. For example, the human skull is on the average 80 times less conductive than the brain and scalp. Therefore, an individual with a 10% thinner skull may result in an 800% change in EEG amplitude across all frequencies. This is one of the reasons that relative measures and ratios are especially important because these measures can naturally correct for amplifier differences and differences in skull thickness.

STATISTICAL FOUNDATIONS: GAUSSIAN DISTRIBUTIONS

The gaussian or normal distribution is a non-linear function that looks like an ideal bell-shaped curve and provides a probability distribution which is symmetrical about its mean. Skewness and kurtosis are measures of the symmetry and peakedness, respectively of the gaussian distribution. In the ideal case of the gaussian distribution, skewness and kurtosis equal zero. In the real world of data sampling distributions, skewness and kurtosis equal to zero is never achieved and, therefore, some reasonable standard of deviation from the ideal is needed in order to determine the approximation of a distribution to gaussian. In the case of the Lifespan EEG database we used the criteria of approximation as a reasonable measure of gaussian distribution. The most serious type of deviation from normality is "skewness" or a unsymmetrical distribution about the mean (e.g., a tail to the left or right of the mean), while the second form of deviation from normality "kurtosis" is the amount of peakedness in the distribution, which is not as serious since the variance is symmetrical about the mean (mean = median). However, it is preferable to attempt to achieve normality as best as one can to insure unbiased estimates of error. The primary reason to achieve "normality" is that the sensitivity of any normative database is determined directly by the shape of the sampling distribution. In a normal distribution, for example, one would expect that five percent of the samples will be equal to or greater than ± 2 standard deviations (SD) and approximately .13% ± 3 SD.

It is important to note that automatic and blindly applied transformations of EEG measures do not insure improved normality of the sampling distribution. For example, it is simple to demonstrate that while some transformations may improve the normality of distributions, these same transforms can also degrade the normality of the distributions. Table 1 shows the effects of transforms on the distributions of the various EEG variables in the lifespan EEG reference normative database. The "No Transform" column shows the deviation from gaussian for the untransformed or raw EEG values and the "Transform" column shows the deviation from gaussian for the transformed EEG values. Table 1 shows that overall the EEG values are well behaved, even without transforms. The only exceptions to this are in EEG phase, total power and absolute power. Transforms of coherence and amplitude asymmetry actually increased skewness or kurtosis, thus blind transformations are not recommended. The asterisks in Table 1 identify which transformed variables are used in the Lifespan EEG normative database. It can be seen that only the transformed EEG phase and the power variables are contained in the database. Table 1 provides the statistics of gaussian distribution of the database. The user of the normative database should take into account the different degrees of gaussian fits of the different variables to understand which variables deviate from normality and to what extent. This information should be used when making clinical evaluations based on the database.

STATISTICAL FOUNDATIONS:
CROSS-VALIDATION

As mentioned in the section on Amplifier and Digital Matching, the statistical accuracy or sensitivity of a normative database is judged

TABLE 1. Gaussian Distribution of the EEG Normative Database

EEG Measure	Skewness		Kurtosis	
	No Transform	Transformed	No Transform	Transformed
Coherence:	0.1%	---	3.8%	---
Delta	0%	---	3.3%	---
Theta	0%	---	2.9%	---
Alpha	0%	---	3.2%	---
Beta	0.2%	---	5.7%	---
Phase (Absolute):	3.2%	0.9%*	27.2%	5.2%*
Delta	2.3%	0.4%*	26.0%	3.6%*
Theta	3.6%	0.5%*	28.9%	3.2%*
Alpha	2.0%	2.1%*	23.0%	8.5%*
Beta	5.0%	0.4%*	31.0%	5.4%*
Amplitude Asym:	0%	---	2.6%	---
Delta	0%	---	2.0%	---
Theta	0%	---	1.7%	---
Alpha	0%	---	3.7%	---
Beta	0%	---	3.0%	---
Relative Power	0%	---	4.5%	2.3%*
Total Power	4.2%	0%*	25.4%	1.8%*
Absolute Power	3.8%	0%*	30.6%	1.8%*

* Transformed variables

directly by the gaussian distribution of the database. The Supreme Court's *Daubert* factor one is met because the gaussian is the null-hypothesis which was tested and factor two will be met by any database because the error estimate was tested and adjusted to approximate a gaussian distribution. *Daubert* factors one and two are expressed as the gaussian sensitivity and accuracy of a database as provided by cross-validation (see Figure 1). There are many different ways to cross-validate a database. One is to obtain independent samples and another is to compute Z-scores for each individual subject in the database. The former is generally not possible because it requires sampling large numbers of additional subjects who have been carefully screened for clinical normality without a history of problems in school, etc. The second method is certainly possible for any database. Cross-validation of the

Lifespan EEG database was accomplished by the latter method in which Z-scores were computed using a leave-one-out procedure for all variables from each individual subject based on his/her respective age-matched mean and SD in the normative database. A distribution of Z-scores for each of the 924 variables for each subject was then tabulated. Table 2 shows the results of the cross-validation of the 625 subjects in the normative EEG database.

A perfect gaussian cross-validation would be 2.3% at + 2 SD, 2.3% at −2 SD, 0.13% at +3 SD and 0.13% at −3 SD. Table 2 shows a cross-validation grand average of 2.58% to 1.98% ± 2 SD and 0.18% to 0.14% ± 3 SD. The Z-score cross-validation results in Table 2 show that the database is statistically accurate and sensitive with slight differences between variables. For example, the power and EEG phase measures showed a small deviation from normality with a tendency toward skewness and kurtosis which is consistent with the values in Table 1.

TABLE 2. Gaussian Cross-Validation of the EEG Normative Database

Measure	% > 2 SD	% < 2 SD	% > 3 SD	% < 3 SD
Delta Amplitude Asym.	2.58	3.08	0.21	0.19
Theta Amplitude Asym.	2.29	2.62	0.15	0.13
Alpha Amplitude Asym.	2.71	2.72	0.18	0.19
Beta Amplitude Asym.	2.68	2.65	0.15	0.15
Delta Coherence	1.99	2.14	0.14	0.22
Theta Coherence	2.22	1.88	0.22	0.16
Alpha Coherence	2.55	1.62	0.18	0.18
Beta Coherence	2.20	1.38	0.18	0.10
Delta Phase †	0.89	3.52	0	0.23
Theta Phase †	1.61	1.87	0.04	0.13
Alpha Phase †	1.61	1.66	0.04	0.24
Beta Phase †	2.83	0.72	0.27	0.03
Absolute Power †	4.15	1.67	0.23	0.12
Relative Power †	4.09	0.52	0.68	0
Total Power †	4.23	1.60	0.08	0.04
Average	2.58	1.98	0.18	0.14

† Data was logged transformed

Figure 3 shows the complex demodulation approximate gaussian distributions in which the transforms or non-transforms in Table 1 were used and the sensitivity calculated as illustrated in Figure 4. Table 3 is an example of a standard Table of Sensitivities for one of the FFT databases.

Figure 4 is an illustrative bell-shaped curve showing the ideal gaussian and the average cross-validation values of the database by which estimates of statistical sensitivity can be derived. True positives equal the percentage of Z-scores that lay within the tails of the gaussian distribution. False negatives (FN) equal the percentage of Z-scores that fall outside of the tails of the gaussian distribution. The error rates or the statistical sensitivity of a quantitative electroencephalogram normative database are directly related to the deviation from a gaussian distribution. Figure 4 depicts a mathematical method of estimating the statistical sensitivity of a normative EEG database in terms of the deviation from gaussian.

Table 3 is an example of the calculated sensitivity of an EEG normative database for different age groups. This same table of sensitivity scores was calculated for the eyes-open, eyes-closed, absolute and relative power in current source density, average reference and linked ears. The percentage of Z-scores in the tails of the gaussian distribution at ± 2 SD for the various databases (LE = linked ears, AVE = average reference and CSD = current source density) are shown in Figures 5 and 6 for the FFT eyes-open and eyes-closed normative databases.

The reliability of different gaussian databases can be measured directly by their deviation from gaussian because the same normative individual subjects are used to validate the different EEG normative databases. For example, average reference norms and current source density norms, when cross-validated using the same subjects as for the linked ears norms gives rise to a reliability coefficient and a statistical reliability reference. The null hypothesis, reliability equals zero, can be directly tested using seven different norms in NeuroGuide.

Figure 7 is an example of visually verifiable reliability and repeatability of the spectra of Z-scores using three different montages (LE, AVE and CSD) derived from the same edited samples of EEG in a traumatic brain injured patient (TBI).

STATISTICAL FOUNDATIONS: VALIDATION BY CLINICAL CORRELATIONS

Validity concerns the relationship between what is being measured and the nature and use to which the measurement is being applied. An-

FIGURE 3. Histograms of the complex demodulation Z-score cross-validation for all ages.

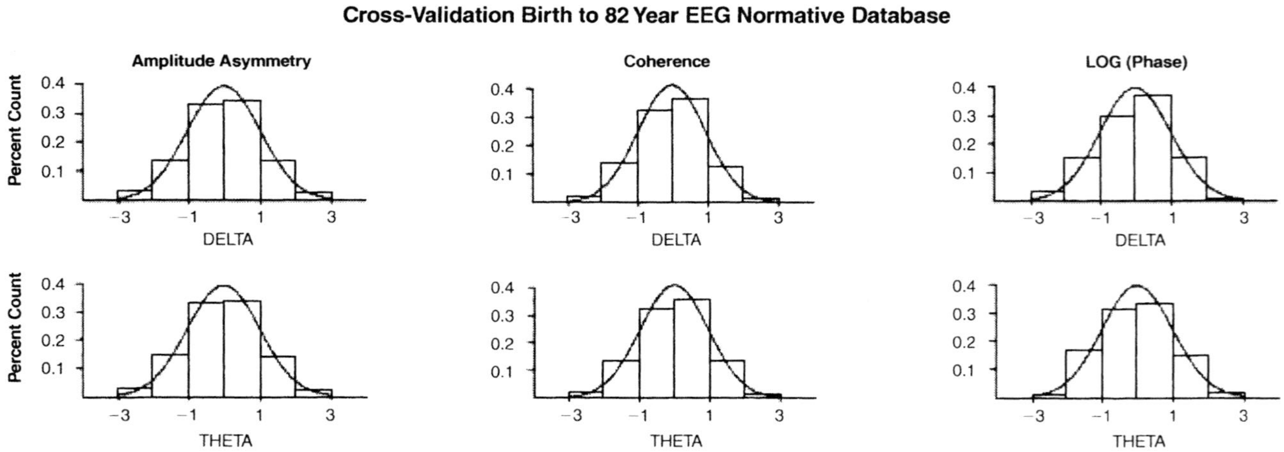

Cross-Validation Birth to 82 Year EEG Normative Database

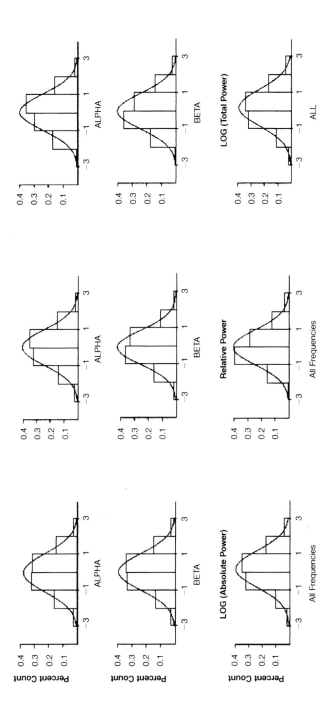

105

FIGURE 4. A normal curve showing values of Z (± 1.96), which includes the proportion which is 0.95 of the total area. The left and right tails of the distribution show probability values of .025 (one-tailed). The results of the cross-validation of 625 subjects showed a classification accuracy that was normally distributed with 2.28% of the Z-scores > ± 2 standard deviations (SD) and 0.16% of the Z-scores > ± 3 SD. The clinical evaluation of EEG measures rely upon such a normal distribution by estimating the probability of finding an observed EEG value in a given range of a normal population and then empirically testing the sensitivity of the database by cross-validation.

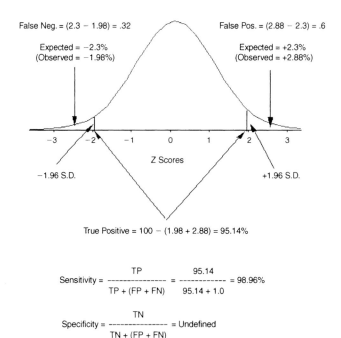

**Sensitivity Based on Deviation from Gaussian
Cross-Validation Accuracy N = 625 Subjects**

other way to put it is that validity is defined as the extent to which any measuring instrument measures what it is intended to measure. Just as reliability is a matter of degree, so is validity. Hypothesis formation and hypothesis testing as emphasized in *Daubert* (1993) is an important part of determining the validity of a scientific measure.

TABLE 3. FFT Normative Database Sensitivities

2 STDEVs	CALC SENSITVITY: FP = TP/(TP + FP) or FN = TP/(TP + FN)			
AGES	(± 2 SD)	(≥ 2 SD)	(≤ −2 SD)	
0-5.99	0.95448265	0.9771774	0.97730526	± **2 Std. Dev.**
6-9.99	0.95440363	0.9772031	0.97720054	
10-12.99	0.9543997	0.97724346	0.97715624	
13-15.99	0.95440512	0.97723601	0.97716911	
16-ADULT	0.9543945	0.97718143	0.97716911	
ALL	0.95442375	0.97720714	0.97721661	

3 STDEVs	CALC SENSITIVITY: FP = TP/(TP + FP) or FN = TP/(TP + FN)			
AGES	(± 3 SD)	(≥ 3 SD)	(≤ −3 SD)	
0-5.99	0.99743898	0.99871123	0.99872774	± **3 Std. Dev.**
6-9.99	0.99744112	0.99871611	0.99872501	
10-12.99	0.99744688	0.99873171	0.99871518	
13-15.99	0.99743186	0.99871951	0.99871237	
16-ADULT	0.99743835	0.99870216	0.99873619	
ALL	0.99744002	0.99871716	0.99872286	

PREDICTIVE VALIDITY
OF A QEEG NORMATIVE DATABASE

Predictive (or criterion) validity has a close relationship to hypothesis testing by subjecting the measure to a discriminant analysis or cluster analysis to some statistical analysis in order to separate a clinical sub-type from a normal reference database. Nunnally (1978) gives a useful definition of predictive validity as, ". . . when the purpose is to use an instrument to estimate some important form of behavior that is external to the measuring instrument itself, the latter being referred to as criterion [predictive] validity." For example, science "validates" the clinical usefulness of a measure by its false positive and false negative rates and by the extent to which there are statistically significant correlations to other clinical measures and, especially, to clinical outcomes.

An example of predictive validity of the linked ears QEEG normative database is shown in Figure 8 in which the normative database was used to discriminate TBI patients from age-matched normal control subjects at a classification accuracy equal to 96.2 (Thatcher et al., 1989). Another example of predictive validity is the ability of QEEG normative values to predict cognitive functioning. Figure 9 shows correlations to full scale IQ as an example of predictive validity and content validity. A more complete analysis of the predictive validity of the normative EEG database is shown in Table 4. In Table 4 the percentage

FIGURE 5. Bar graphs of percentage deviation of Z-scores from the ideal gaussian cross-validation in eyes-closed linked ears, average reference and current source density norms.

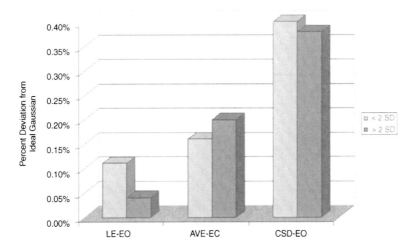

FIGURE 6. Bar graphs of the percentage deviation from the ideal gaussian cross-validation in the eyes-open condition linked ears, average reference and current source density norms.

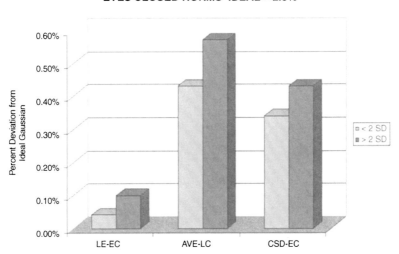

FIGURE 7. Example of reliability between different normative databases and montages in a TBI patient. The general spectral shape is consistently present while the magnitude of deviation from normal and the spatial localization of the deviation increased from linked ears to average reference to current source density (CSD).

Linked Ears

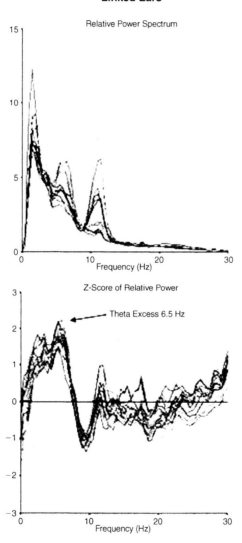

FIGURE 7 (continued)

Average Reference

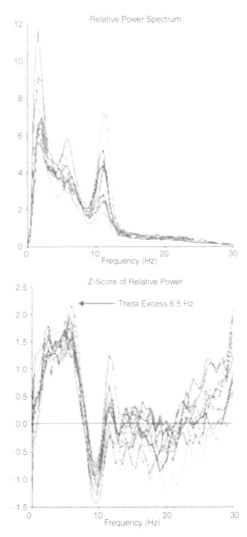

Current Source Density

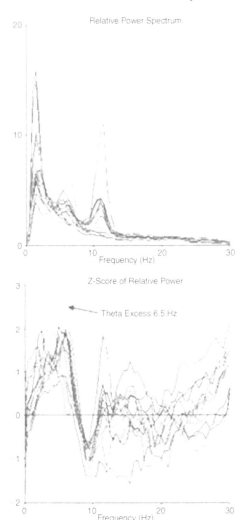

FIGURE 8. Example of a typical scattergram in the content and predictive validation step in Figure 1. The y-axis is full scale IQ and the x-axis is amplitude asymmetry ([(R + L/R − L) × 200], see Thatcher et al., 1983 for further details). The correlation between IQ and amplitude asymmetry in this example was r = 0.460, N = 466 and P < .0001.

Example of Content Validity of EEG Norms
Scatterplots of Amp. Asymmetry with IQ & School Achievement Tests Measures P < .0001

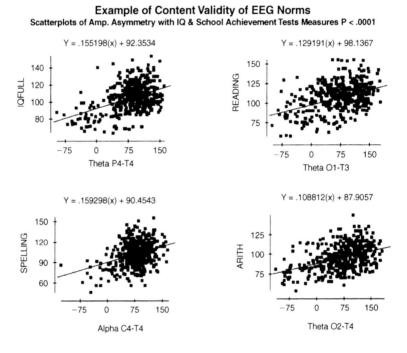

of statistically significant correlations at P < .01 between QEEG, normative EEG, and WRAT school achievement scores and measures of intelligence are shown.

EXAMPLES OF CONTENT VALIDITY
OF A QEEG NORMATIVE DATABASE

Content validity is defined by the extent to which an empirical measurement reflects a specific domain of content. For example, a test in arithmetic operations would not be content valid if the test problems focused only on addition, thus neglecting subtraction, multiplication and division. By the same token, a content-valid measure of cognitive decline following a stroke should include measures of memory capacity, attention and executive function, etc.

FIGURE 9. An example of the normative database predictive validity as demonstrated in a discriminant analysis of 264 mild traumatic brain injured patients and 108 age-matched normal control subjects (Thatcher et al., 1989). The discriminant accuracy, upon replication, was > 95%.

Montage: LINKEARS   EEG ID: Demo1

Traumatic Brain Injury Discriminant Analysis

TBI DISCRIMINANT SCORE = 0.53   TBI PROBABILITY INDEX = 99.0%

The TBI Probability Index is the subject's probability of membership in the mild traumatic brain injury population (see Thatcher et al., EEG and Clin. Neurophysiol., 73: 93-106, 1989).

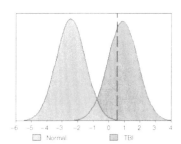

			RAW	Z
FP1-F3	COH	Theta	82.41	0.49
T3-T5	COH	Beta	71.81	1.64
C3-P3	COH	Beta	82.19	1.38
FP2-F4	PHA	Beta	0.11	-1.16
F3-F4	PHA	Beta	0.16	-1.26
F4-T6	AMP	Beta	3.67	1.22
F8-T6	AMP	Alpha	-57.85	1.25
F4-T6	AMP	Alpha	35.04	1.02
F8-T6	AMP	Beta	9.93	1.68
F3-O1	AMP	Alpha	-75.59	0.44
F4-O2	AMP	Alpha	-88.52	0.25
F7-O1	AMP	Alpha	120.33	-0.49
F4-02	AMP	Beta	-36.64	0.19
P3	RP	Alpha	29.91	-1.29
P4	RP	Alpha	31.14	-1.16
O1	RP	Alpha	40.26	-1.03
O2	RP	Alpha	43.11	-0.90
T4	RP	Alpha	21.37	-1.19
T5	RP	Alpha	29.34	-1.20
T6	RP	Alpha	31.69	-1.21

TBI SEVERITY INDEX = 4.91

This severity score places the patient in the MODERATE range of severity.

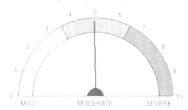

			RAW	Z
FP1-C3	COH	Delta	56.57	0.96
FP1-FP2	COH	Theat	95.12	1.62
O1-F7	COH	Alpha	9.94	-1.14
O2-T6	COH	Alpha	85.79	0.46
P3-O1	COH	Beta	85.04	1.57
FP1-T3	PHA	Theta	-1.63	-0.83
T3-T4	PHA	Theta	3.94	-1.20
O1-F7	PHA	Alpha	7.73	-1.80
F7-F8	PHA	Alpha	1.87	-0.03
T5-T6	PHA	Beta	1.06	-0.88
C3-F7	AMP	Delta	20.73	-1.32
FP2-F4	AMP	Delta	-18.93	0.14
C4F8	AMP	Delta	11.10	-1.55
O1-O2	AMP	Theta	4.12	0.36
P3-F7	AMP	Alpha	79.66	-1.51
FP2-P4	AMP	Alpha	-74.49	0.96

The TBI Severity Index is an estimate of the neurological severity of injury (see Thatcher et al., J Neuropsychiatry and Clinical Neuoscience, 13(1): 77-87, 2001).

TABLE 4. Effect Size: QEEG Measures with School Achievement Tests and IQ Measures Percent Significant Correlations at P ≤ .01, N = 466

Amplitude Asymmetry

P ≤ .01	READING	SPELLING	ARITH	IQFULL	IQVERB	IQPERF
DELTA	64%	61%	55%	64%	61%	61%
THETA	78%	70%	70%	70%	67%	59%
ALPHA	63%	63%	53%	64%	63%	52%
BETA	56%	56%	34%	58%	61%	47%

Coherence

P ≤ .01	READING	SPELLING	ARITH	IQFULL	IQVERB	IQPERF
DELTA	27%	14%	41%	38%	22%	38%
THETA	27%	6%	36%	30%	27%	23%
ALPHA	9%	6%	45%	11%	14%	5%
BETA	11%	5%	38%	22%	17%	6%

Absolute Phase

P ≤ .01	READING	SPELLING	ARITH	IQFULL	IQVERB	IQPERF
DELTA	11%	8%	8%	16%	6%	17%
THETA	9%	5%	8%	13%	9%	17%
ALPHA	9%	3%	33%	14%	19%	6%
BETA	9%	5%	30%	6%	9%	3%

Relative Power

P ≤ .01	READING	SPELLING	ARITH	IQFULL	IQVERB	IQPERF
DELTA	13%	0%	31%	0%	6%	0%
THETA	56%	44%	94%	6%	6%	0%
ALPHA	19%	0%	75%	0%	0%	0%
BETA	13%	6%	44%	19%	13%	13%

Relative Power Ratios

P ≤ .01	READING	SPELLING	ARITH	IQFULL	IQVERB	IQPERF
Theta/Beta	50%	44%	63%	56%	56%	50%
Theta/Alpha	13%	0%	69%	0%	0%	0%
Alpha/Beta	50%	31%	50%	38%	38%	25%
Delta/Theta	19%	25%	56%	19%	13%	25%

There are many examples of the clinical content validity of QEEG and normative databases in ADD, ADHD, schizophrenia, compulsive disorders, depression, epilepsy, TBI (Thatcher, Bivier, McAlaster, & Salazar,1998; Thatcher, Biver, Camacho, McAlaster, & Salazar, 1998) and a wide number of clinical groupings of patients as reviewed by Hughes and John (1999). There are over 280 citations in the review by Hughes and John and there are approximately twenty-three citations to peer-reviewed journal articles in which a normal reference database was used. A year 2003 internet search of the National Library of Medicine will give citations to many more QEEG and content validity peer-reviewed studies using a reference normal group than were included in the Hughes and John review.

NON-PARAMETRIC STATISTICS TO MEASURE CONTENT VALIDITY OF A QEEG NORMATIVE DATABASE

Non-parametric statistics such as the binomial probability and for small sample sizes the Poisson probability are simple non-parametric tests that are distribution free and automatically adjust for multiple comparisons. The catch is that the non-parametric statistics must define a hypothesis by a specific statistical probability alpha level; otherwise they do not work. The binomial distribution is defined as $P(X) = \binom{N}{x} p^x (1 - p)^{N-x}$ of successful outcomes at a specific probability; for example, P < .01 for a specific hypothesis. N equals the number of Z-tests, p is the 'yes' and q the 'no' test of the null hypothesis, r is the alpha cut-off for the probability (e.g., P < .01). For example, the null hypothesis is that by chance there will be one event per 64 observations at P < .01. The experiment is run and there were 50 observations at P < .01. The exact probability for the binomial equation in this instance is probability $P(X) = .0000060$.

Figure 10 is an example of the statistical significance of some of the clinical correlations of the EEG database (i.e., Wide Range Achievement Test for Reading, Spelling, Arithmetic and Full Scale IQ). E(X) is the expected number of correlations at P < .01. X equals the number of observed correlations at P < .01 and P(X) equals the binomial probability to reject the null hypothesis. Table 4 shows the observed percentage of correlations at P < .01 by which the X value in Figure 10 corresponds.

FIGURE 10. An example of the use of the non-parametric statistic of the binomial probability distribution to calculate the alpha level for the content validation of clinical measures with the QEEG normative database. The binomial probability is defined as $P(X) = \binom{N}{x}p^x(1 - p)^{N-x}$ of successful outcomes defined as a correlation coefficient at the probability of P < .01. N = the total number of correlations for a given QEEG measure, X = the number of observed correlations at P .01; E(X) = the number of expected correlations at P < .01. P(X) = the distribution free binomial probabilities. The percentage of statistically significant correlations at P < .01 is shown in Table 4.

BINOMIAL PROBABILITIES of Expected Significant Correlations
qEEG Measures with School Achievement Tests & IQ Measures, @ P <=.01

Amplitude Asymmetry			Reading		Spelling		Arithmetic		IQ FULL	
P <= .01	N	E(X)	X	P(X)	X	P(X)	X	P(X)	X	P(X)
DELTA	64	1	41	0.0000	39	0.0000	35	0.0000	41	0.0000
THETA	64	1	50	0.0000	45	0.0000	45	0.0000	45	0.0000
ALPHA	64	1	40	0.0000	40	0.0000	34	0.0000	41	0.0000
BETA	64	1	36	0.0000	36	0.0000	22	0.0000	37	0.0000

Coherence			Reading		Spelling		Arithmetic		IQ FULL	
P <= .01	N	E(X)	X	P(X)	X	P(X)	X	P(X)	X	P(X)
DELTA	64	1	17	0.0000	9	0.0000	26	0.0000	24	0.0000
THETA	64	1	17	0.0000	4	0.0005	23	0.0000	19	0.0000
ALPHA	64	1	6	0.0000	4	0.0005	29	0.0000	7	0.0000
BETA	64	1	7	0.0000	3	0.0039	24	0.0000	14	0.0000

Absolute Phase			Reading		Spelling		Arithmetic		IQ FULL	
P <= .01	N	E(X)	X	P(X)	X	P(X)	X	P(X)	X	P(X)
DELTA	64	1	7	0.0000	5	0.0000	5	0.0000	10	0.0000
THETA	64	1	6	0.0000	3	0.0039	5	0.0000	8	0.0000
ALPHA	64	1	6	0.0000	2	0.0265	21	0.0000	9	0.0000
BETA	64	1	6	0.0000	3	0.0039	19	0.0000	4	0.0005

Relative Power			Reading		Spelling		Arithmetic		IQ FULL	
P <= .01	N	E(X)	X	P(X)	X	P(X)	X	P(X)	X	P(X)
DELTA	16	0	2	0.0005	0	0.1485	5	0.0000	0	0.1485
THETA	16	0	9	0.0000	7	0.0000	15	0.0000	1	0.0109
ALPHA	16	0	3	0.0000	0	0.1485	12	0.0000	0	0.1485
BETA	16	0	2	0.0005	1	0.0109	7	0.0000	3	0.0000

Relative Power Ratios			Reading		Spelling		Arithmetic		IQ FULL	
P <= .01	N	E(X)	X	P(X)	X	P(X)	X	P(X)	X	P(X)
Theta/Beta	16	0	8	0.0000	7	0.0000	10	0.0000	9	0.0000
Theta/Alpha	16	0	2	0.0005	0	0.1485	11	0.0000	0	0.1485
Alpha/Beta	16	0	8	0.0000	5	0.0000	8	0.0000	6	0.0000
Delta/Theta	16	0	3	0.0000	4	0.0000	9	0.0000	3	0.0000

EFFECT SIZE OF A NORMATIVE EEG DATABASE

The effect size of a normative database for any set of clinical measures can be estimated from the percentage of statistically significant correlations (Cohen, 1977). Table 4 effect sizes are based on the percentage of statistically significant observations at alpha set at P < .01. Based on the percentage in Table 4, one can translate the number in column X in Figure 9 as the number observed out of a total universe of correlations. It can be seen that amplitude asymmetry and ratios of power have the strongest effect size, especially in arithmetic and IQ. The peer-reviewed literature clearly demonstrates that QEEG is clinically valid with varying effect sizes (Hughes & John, 1999). Estimates of effect size are relative clinical validation measures that a clinician or scientist takes into consideration when rendering a clinical or scientific judgment. Effect size is also useful in counseling graduate students to calculate the sample size that they will need in their thesis by power analysis.

NON-PARAMETRIC STATISTICS, ESTIMATES OF ALPHA LEVELS AND THE ISSUE OF MULTIPLE COMPARISONS IN A SINGLE SUBJECT COMPARISON TO AN EEG NORMATIVE DATABASE

The use of many t-tests or Z-tests in EEG applications requires some adjustment for the total number of tests in order to accurately estimate levels of alpha or the probability of a Type I error (i.e., saying something is statistically significant when it is not). As explained by Hayes (1973), multiple comparisons refers to multiple group comparisons and not to the adjustment of the total number of t-tests or Z-tests, whereas non-parametric statistics is one of the best methods to adjust for both Type I and Type II error rates.

Figure 11 shows an example of the use of the binomial probability distribution to determine the alpha level for a single subject's comparison to the complex demodulation normative database. The number of Z-tests is represented as 'N,' E(X) equals the number expected by chance alone at P < .05 (top of Figure 10) or at P < .01 (bottom of Figure 11). X equals the number of successful Z-tests observed and P(X) equals the binomial probability.

Figure 11 is only one example of how non-parametric statistics can be used to eliminate multiple comparison problems.

FIGURE 11. An example of the use of the non-parametric statistic of the binomial probability distribution to calculate the alpha level for the complex demodulation norms for a given patient. The binomial probability is defined as $P(X) = \binom{N}{x}p^x(1 - p)^{N-x}$ of successful outcomes at the probability of P < .05 and P < .01. N = the total number of Z-scores in the measure set, X = the number of observed Z-scores at P < .05 and P .01; E(X) = the number of expected Z-scores at P < .05 or at the probability P < .01.

Z <=−1.96 or Z >= 1.96 @ .05 Significance Level

EEG by Frequency			Delta		Theta		Alpha		Beta	
P(at least X)	N	E(X)	X	P(X)	X	P(X)	X	P(X)	X	P(X)
Relative Power	16	1	2	0.0429	13	0.0000	0	0.5599	0	0.5599
Amplitude Asymmetry	64	3	0	0.9625	1	0.8361	0	0.9625	0	0.9625
Coherence	64	3	9	0.0012	17	0.0000	2	0.6265	5	0.1001
Phase	64	3	7	0.0142	1	0.8361	0	0.9625	1	0.8361

EEG by Hemisphere			Intra LEFT		Intra RIGHT		Per EEG		Overall EEG	
P(at least X)	N	E(X)	X	P(X)	X	P(X)	X	P(X)	X	P(X)
Relative Power	37	2	6	0.0009	9	0.0000	15	0.0000	58	0.0052
Amplitude Asymmetry	112	6	1	0.9779	0	0.9968	1	1.0000	N=832	
Coherence	112	6	18	0.0000	12	0.0040	33	0.0000	E(X)=42	
Phase	112	6	3	0.8165	4	0.6641	9	0.8274		

Z <=−2.576 or Z >= 2.576 @ .01 Significance Level

EEG by Frequency			Delta		Theta		Alpha		Beta	
P(at least X)	N	E(X)	X	P(X)	X	P(X)	X	P(X)	X	P(X)
Relative Power	16	0	0	0.1485	6	0.0000	0	0.1485	0	0.1485
Amplitude Asymmetry	64	1	0	0.4744	0	0.4744	0	0.4744	0	0.4744
Coherence	64	1	1	0.1346	2	0.0265	0	0.4744	0	0.4744
Phase	64	1	0	0.4744	0	0.4744	0	0.4744	0	0.4744

EEG by Hemisphere			Intra LEFT		Intra RIGHT		Per EEG		Overall EEG	
P(at least X)	N	E(X)	X	P(X)	X	P(X)	X	P(X)	X	P(X)
Relative Power	32	0	3	0.0003	3	0.0003	6	0.0000	9	0.3233
Amplitude Asymmetry	112	1	0	0.6756	0	0.6756	0	0.9237	N=832	
Coherence	112	1	3	0.0265	0	0.6756	3	0.2548	E(X)=8	
Phase	112	1	0	0.6756	0	0.6756	0	0.9237		

PEER REVIEWED PUBLICATIONS
AND INDEPENDENT REPLICATIONS

The University of Maryland NeuroGuide EEG database presented in this paper is unique and represents a sample or a "snapshot" of electrical events in a medium-size population. The oldest person in the database is age 82, but the sample size from age 50 to 100 needs to be expanded as the population grows older. Each normative EEG database is necessarily unique by virtue of subject selection, number of subjects, age span and arrangement of the subjects and the digital methods. Also, each EEG database uses different methods to acquire the EEG and to edit and analyze the EEG. In order to use any EEG normative database matching amplifiers and analytic methods must first be accomplished.

Independent replication of certain aspects of the NeuroGuide University of Maryland EEG Database (Thatcher et al., 1983, 1986, 1987; Thatcher, 1998) have been published and they are consistent with the NYU School of Medicine database (i.e., John et al., 1987) and the Harvard School of Medicine database (i.e., Duffy et al., 1994). Also, most of the acquisition methods, analysis methods and results of experiments using the University of Maryland EEG database in this paper and the NYU and Harvard databases have been published in refereed journals which are cited below. Aspects of the development of relative power of the University of Maryland NeuroGuide EEG norms have been replicated in studies by Matousek and Petersen (1973) as analyzed by John et al. (1977), Fischer (1987), Thatcher (1980), Epstein (1980), van Baal (1997), Hanlon (1996) and Hanlon, Thatcher, and Cline (1999). Aspects of the EEG coherence development in the database presented in this paper have been replicated by Gasser, Verleger, Bacher, and Stroka (1988), Gasser, Jennen-Steinmetz, Stroka, Verleger, and Mocks (1998), Thatcher, Biver, Camacho, McAlaster, and Salazar (1998) and by van Baal and others in genetic analysis (van Beijsterveldt, Molenaar, de Geus, & Boomsma, 1996; van Baal, 1997; van Ball, de Geus, & Boomsma, 1998; van Beijsterveldt, Molenaar, de Geus, & Boomsma, 1998).

REFERENCES

Bendat, J. S., & Piersol, A. G. (1980). *Engineering applications of correlation and spectral analysis*. New York: John Wiley & Sons.

Cohen, J. (1977). *Statistical power analysis for the behavioral sciences*. New York: Academic Press.

Daubert v. Merrell Dow Pharmaceuticals (Daubert), 61 U.S.L.W 4805 (U.S. June 29, 1993).

Duffy, F., Hughes, J. R., Miranda, F., Bernad, P., & Cook, P. (1994). Status of quantitative EEG (QEEG) in clinical practice. *Clinical Electroencephalography, 25* (4), VI-XXII.

Epstein, H. T. (1980). EEG developmental stages. *Developmental Psychobiology, 13,* 629-631.

Fischer, K. W. (1987). Relations between brain and cognitive development. *Child Development, 57,* 623-632.

Gasser, T., Verleger, R., Bacher, P., & Sroka, L. (1988). Development of the EEG of school-age children and adolescents. I. Analysis of band power. *Electroencephalography and Clinical Neurophysiology, 69* (2), 91-99.

Gasser, T., Jennen-Steinmetz, C., Sroka, L., Verleger, R., & Mocks, J. (1988). Development of the EEG of school-age children and adolescents. II: Topography. *Electroencephalography Clinical Neurophysiology, 69* (2), 100-109.

Hanlon, H. W. (1996). Topographically different regional networks impose structural limitations on both sexes in early postnatal development. In: K. Pribram & J. King (Eds.), *Learning as self-organization* (pp. 311-376). Mahwah, NJ: Lawrence Erlbaum Assoc., Inc.

Hanlon, H. W., Thatcher, R. W., & Cline, M. J. (1999). Gender differences in the development of EEG coherence in normal children. *Developmental Neuropsychology, 16* (3), 479-506.

Hayes, W. L. (1973). *Statistics for the social sciences.* New York: Holt, Rhinehart and Winston.

Hughes, J. R., & John, E. R. (1999). Conventional and quantitative electroencephalography in psychiatry. *Neuropsychiatry, 11,* 190-208.

John, E. R., Karmel, B., Corning, W., Easton, P., Brown, D., Ahn, H. et al. (1977). Neurometrics: Numerical taxonomy identifies different profiles of brain functions within groups of behaviorally similar people. *Science, 196,* 1393-1410.

John, E. R., Prichep, L. S., & Easton, P. (1987). Normative data banks and neurometrics: Basic concepts, methods and results of norm construction. In A. Remond (Ed.), *Handbook of electroencephalography and clinical neurophysiology: Vol. III. Computer analysis of the EEG and other neurophysiological signals* (pp. 449-495). Amsterdam: Elsevier.

John, E. R., Prichep, L. S., Fridman, J., & Easton, P. (1988). Neurometrics: Computer assisted differential diagnosis of brain dysfunctions. *Science, 293,* 162-169.

Kaiser, D. A., & Sterman, M. B. (2001). Automatic artifact detection, overlapping windows and state transitions. *Journal of Neurotherapy, 4* (3), 85-92.

Mahle, S. (2001). *Daubert* and the Law and Science of Expert Testimony in Business Litigation. *Business litigation in Florida* (4th ed.). Tallahassee, FL: Florida Bar Association.

Matousek, M., & Petersen, I. (1973). Frequency analysis of the EEG background activity by means of age dependent EEG quotients. In P. Kellaway & I. Petersen (Eds.), *Automation of clinical electroencephalography* (pp. 75-102). New York: Raven Press.

Nunnally, J.C. (1978). *Psychometric theory.* New York: McGraw-Hill.

Otnes, R. K., & Enochson, L. (1972). *Digital time series analysis.* New York: John Wiley & Sons.

Press, W. H., Teukolsky, S. A., Vettering, W. T., & Flannery, B. P. (1994). *Numerical recipes in C.* Cambridge, UK: Cambridge University Press.

Pascual-Marqui, R. D., Gonzalez-Andino, S. L., Valdes-Sosa, P. A., & Biscay-Lirio, R. (1988). Current source density estimation and interpolation based on spherical harmonic Fourier expansion. *International Journal of Neuroscience, 43,* 237-249.

Thatcher, R. W. (1980). Neurolinguistics: Theoretical and evolutionary perspectives. *Brain and Language, 11,* 235-260.

Thatcher, R. W., Lester, M. L., McAlaster, R., & Horst, R. (1982). Effects of low levels of cadmium and lead on cognitive functioning in children. *Archives of Environmental Health, 37,* 159-166.

Thatcher, R. W., McAlaster, R., Lester, M. L., Horst, R. L., & Cantor, D. S. (1983). Hemispheric EEG asymmetries related to cognitive functioning in children. In A. Perecuman (Ed.), *Cognitive processing in the right hemisphere* (pp. 125-145). New York: Academic Press.

Thatcher, R. W., & Krause, P. (1986). Corticocortical association fibers and EEG coherence: A two compartmental model. *Electroencephalography and Clinical Neurophysiology, 64,* 123-143.

Thatcher, R. W., Walker, R. A., & Guidice, S. (1987). Human cerebral hemispheres develop at different rates and ages. *Science, 236,* 1110-1113.

Thatcher, R. W., Walker, R. A., Gerson, I., & Geisler, F. (1989). EEG discriminant analyses of mild head trauma. *Electroencephalography and Clinical Neurophysiology, 73,* 93-106.

Thatcher, R. W. (1991). Maturation of the human frontal lobes: Physiological evidence for staging. *Developmental Neuropsychology, 7* (3), 370-394.

Thatcher, R. W. (1992). Cyclic cortical reorganization during early childhood. *Brain and Cognition, 20,* 24-50.

Thatcher, R. W. (1994). Psychopathology of early frontal lobe damage: Dependence on cycles of postnatal development. *Developmental Pathology, 6,* 565-596.

Thatcher, R. W. (1998). EEG normative databases and EEG biofeedback. *Journal of Neurotherapy, 2* (4), 8-39.

Thatcher, R. W., Biver, C., McAlaster, R., & Salazar, A. M. (1998). Biophysical linkage between MRI and EEG coherence in traumatic brain injury. *NeuroImage, 8* (4), 307-326.

Thatcher, R. W., Biver, C., Camacho, M., McAlaster, R., & Salazar, A. M. (1998). Biophysical linkage between MRI and EEG amplitude in traumatic brain injury. *NeuroImage, 7,* 352-367.

Thatcher, R. W., Biver, C., & North, D. (2003). Quantitative EEG and the Frye and Daubert Standards of Admissibility. *Clinical Electroencephalography, 34* (2), 39-53.

van Baal, G. C. (1997). A genetic perspective on the developing brain: EEG indices of neural functioning in five to seven year old twins. *Organization for scientific research (NWO).* The Netherlands: Vrije University Press.

van Baal, G. C., de Geus, E. J., & Boomsma, D. I. (1998). Genetic influences on EEG coherence in 5-year-old twins. *Behavioral Genetics, 28* (1), 9-19.

van Beijsterveldt, C. E., Molenaar, P. C., de Geus, E. J., & Boomsma, D. I. (1996). Heritability of human brain functioning as assessed by electroencephalography. *American Journal of Human Genetics, 58* (3), 562-573.

van Beijsterveldt, C. E., Molenaar, P. C., de Geus, E. J., & Boomsma, D. I. (1998). Genetic and environmental influences on EEG coherence. *Behavioral Genetics, 28* (6), 443-453.

Comparison of QEEG Reference Databases in Basic Signal Analysis and in the Evaluation of Adult ADHD

J. Noland White, PhD

SUMMARY. *Introduction.* Despite the relatively widespread investigation of potential quantitative electroencephalographic (QEEG) characteristics of childhood attention deficit hyperactivity disorder (ADHD), relatively little is known about the possible QEEG characteristics of adult ADHD. In addition to general magnitude or power measures, or ratios of these measures, the additional analyses and comparisons provided by QEEG reference databases may prove useful in providing unique markers for adult ADHD.

Method. This investigation reports the findings of evaluations using three QEEG reference databases for a sample of ten adults previously di-

J. Noland White is Assistant Professor of Psychology, Department of Psychology, CBX 90, Georgia College and State University, Milledgeville, GA 31061 (E-mail: noland.white@gcsu.edu).

The author wants to thank Joel F. Lubar for his encouragement and support throughout this project. The author offers special thanks to Leslie Sherlin and Efthymios Angelakis for their assistance and contributions to this study.

The author also wants to thank the following individuals for making available the products used in this study: Lexicor Health Systems for the data acquisition equipment, William J. Hudspeth for the NeuroRep QEEG Analysis and Report System, M. Barry Sterman and David A. Kaiser for the SKIL Topometric Software package, and Marco Congedo and Leslie Sherlin of NovaTech EEG for the EEG Editor and EureKa3! QEEG analysis package.

agnosed with ADHD. The packages used in the current investigation included the NeuroRep QEEG Analysis and Report System, the SKIL Topometric QEEG software package, and the NovaTech EEG EureKa3! QEEG analysis package.

Results. As compared with the respective databases, adults with ADHD appear to demonstrate higher levels of 8-10 Hz activity during both eyes-closed and eyes-open resting baselines. They also appear to demonstrate frontal involvement as evidenced by hypercoherence and hypercomodulation in frontal areas.

Conclusions. Each of the three QEEG reference databases appears to offer unique markers for adult ADHD. However, other apparent differences were found to be attributable to specific analysis packages rather than the clinical group itself. An investigation of basic signal analyses also revealed differences between the three packages. Results of the respective analyses and possible implications are discussed. *[Article copies available for a fee from The Haworth Document Delivery Service: 1-800-HAWORTH. E-mail address: <docdelivery@haworthpress.com> Website: <http://www.HaworthPress.com> © 2003 by The Haworth Press, Inc. All rights reserved.]*

KEYWORDS. Attention deficit hyperactivity disorder (ADHD), quantitative electroencephalography, QEEG, assessment, coherence, comodulation, database, LORETA

INTRODUCTION

The utility of quantitative electroencephalography (QEEG) in the diagnosis of childhood attention deficit hyperactivity disorder (ADHD) has been explored for over a quarter of a century. Some consistencies have been noted such as increased theta activity in frontal or central regions (Barry, Clarke, & Johnstone, 2003; Chabot & Serfontein, 1996; Clarke, Barry, McCarthy, & Selikowitz, 1998; Mann, Lubar, Zimmerman, Miller, & Muenchen, 1992; Monastra, Lubar, & Linden, 2001; Monastra et al., 1999) or deficits in alpha or beta activity (Barry et al., 2003; Clarke et al., 1998; Mann et al., 1992). Despite these apparent consistencies in children, it has recently been suggested that EEG variability exists and that there may be additional clusters of activity or QEEG-defined subtypes of ADHD (Barry et al., 2003; Chabot & Serfontein, 1996; Clarke et al., 1998; Clarke, Barry, McCarthy, & Selikowitz, 2001).

Although ADHD may persist into adulthood, the QEEG literature is relatively sparse with regard to investigations of adults with ADHD. Some literature has suggested that adult ADHD is characterized by some of the same QEEG features as childhood ADHD such as an increased theta/low-beta ratio (Monastra et al., 1999). Other research suggests that the increased theta is maintained but without beta deficits (Bresnahan, Anderson, & Barry, 1999; Bresnahan & Barry, 2002).

QEEG variables have also been examined in conjunction with neuropsychological task performance. In a recent study of adult college students, approximately 50% of the ADHD sample demonstrated greater impairment than their ADHD colleagues as evidenced by at least two of the three attention quotient scores on the Intermediate Visual and Auditory Continuous Performance Test (IVA; White, 2001). Furthermore, these same individuals with greater impairment on the IVA demonstrated significantly higher theta/low-beta power ratios at a fronto-central location (Fz) as compared with their ADHD colleagues during two other neuropsychological tasks, the Paced Auditory Serial Addition Task (PASAT) and the Wisconsin Card Sorting Test (WCST; White, 2001).

Additionally, as compared with a group of non-clinical controls, the adults with ADHD demonstrated higher levels of low-alpha (8-10 Hz) or high-alpha (10-12 Hz) activity, depending on the task condition (White, 2001). Although this study had a small number of clinical individuals ($n = 10$), these findings, coupled with the aforementioned studies, speak to potential diversity in the QEEG characteristics of adult ADHD. Consequently, just as research has indicated that childhood ADHD may be characterized by more than one pattern of QEEG activity, there is a need for further investigation of possible quantitative electroencephalographic variations in adults with ADHD.

One method used to identify potentially pathognomic QEEG variations is the incorporation of a QEEG reference database. There are several such databases commercially available, but to date, a comparison of databases has not been performed in the attempt to identify specific QEEG features which may be specific to a given clinical population such as adults with ADHD. Accordingly, to further evaluate the ADHD subjects from the White (2001) study, the current investigation will compare the results of analyses from three such databases. The databases used in the study are those associated with the NeuroRep QEEG Analysis and Report System (version 4; Hudspeth, 2000), the SKIL Topometric Software Package (version 2.05; Sterman & Kaiser, 2000), and the EureKa3! Quantitative EEG Analysis System (version 3.0; Congedo, 2002a).

EXPERIMENT 1

Method

Before using each of the database packages to evaluate the adult ADHD participants, standardized files were submitted to each software package to investigate potential differences between the programs themselves that might affect the interpretation of the clinical analyses. As such, three data files were created for this part of the study.

The first file was generated through the use of an external signal generator and recorded with a Lexicor NeuroSearch-24 system using Lexicor NeuroLex (v1.51) acquisition software. The second file was also generated with the same external signal generator but recorded with NeuroLex (v41E) acquisition software. Lastly, a third file was digitally created with the WaveGeneratore (Congedo, 2002b) software package. All three files were comprised of a 10 Hz, 20 μv peak amplitude sinusoidal signal at channels Fz, Cz, and Pz, with a sampling rate of 128 K. The three files will be subsequently referred to as v151, v41E, and digital, respectively. All three signal files were analyzed with both NeuroRep and EureKa3!; Lexicor v41E files are not compatible with SKIL, thus the v41E file was not submitted to SKIL.

Results

Following analysis with each package, spectral amplitudes were obtained from their respective output sources (NeuroRep *.FTA output file; SKIL spectral value grid; EureKa3! spectral amplitude output file). The spectral amplitude results from all three analyses are found in Table 1.

Although visual inspection of the 10 Hz spectral amplitude values revealed an obvious difference between programs, planned statistical analysis consisted of a one-way analysis of variance (ANOVA). As such, the 10 Hz spectral amplitudes, across sites (Fz, Cz, Pz), for the v151 and digital files were analyzed with a one-way ANOVA. The one-way ANOVA revealed that reported 10 Hz spectral amplitudes did in fact differ significantly as a function of analysis program, $F(2, 15) = 845.99$, $p < .001$.

TABLE 1. Results of 10 Hz, 20 µv Signal File Analysis

	v151*			v41E*			Digital*		
	Fz	*Cz*	*Pz*	*Fz*	*Cz*	*Pz*	*Fz*	*Cz*	*Pz*
NeuroRep	17.39	19.9	18.6	17.3	19.7	18.5	19.4	19.4	19.4
SKIL	41.3	46.7	43.9	NA	NA	NA	40.0	40.0	40.0
EureKa3!	2.18	2.47	2.3	2.16	2.44	2.30	2.23	2.23	2.23

*Original signal was 10 Hz, 20 µv; reported values are absolute 10 Hz amplitude in microvolts (µv)

The reported spectral amplitudes for the NeuroRep analysis (M = 19.02, SD = .90) were closest to the original file parameters. Both the SKIL (M = 41.98, SD = 2.76) and EureKa3! (M = 2.27, SD = .10) spectral amplitude values were different from the original signal parameters.

Given the possibility that individual program features such as windowing and scaling factors may influence a single-frequency sine wave differently than mixed EEG signals, an additional comparison was made by evaluating one of the control subject's eyes-closed baseline data (recorded with Lexicor NeuroLex v151). For each of the three programs, the spectral amplitudes were examined for the 4 Hz, 8 Hz, 12 Hz, 16 Hz, and 20 Hz bins. Those values are reported in Table 2. In general, the reported spectral amplitudes appeared to be more similar for the NeuroRep and EureKa3! results whereas the SKIL results were of larger amplitude.

Discussion

In sum, Experiment 1 revealed that all three packages report different values for spectral amplitudes when compared with data files of known parameters. NeuroRep reported values that were most similar to the original data parameters whereas the values reported for both SKIL and EureKa3! were quite different. When an actual subject data file was analyzed, again, different spectral amplitudes were reported for the three programs.

There are likely two primary causes for the observed differences. The first being variations in reference or montage because different montages produce different voltage values (Fisch, 1999; Niedermeyer, 1999). Both NeuroRep and SKIL use a linked ear reference whereas EureKa3! uses an average reference. The other likely cause is inter-program differences in windowing and scaling factors. Windowing causes

TABLE 2. Results of Eyes-Closed Baseline Spectral Analyses for Single Control Subject

	4 Hz*			8 Hz*			12 Hz*			16 Hz*			20 Hz*		
	Fz	Cz	Pz	Fz	Cz	Pz	Fz	Cz	Pz	Fz	Cz	Pz	Fz	Cz	Pz
NeuroRep	1.16	1.36	1.44	2.9	3.78	5.48	1.02	1.17	1.58	0.74	0.84	0.83	0.56	0.66	0.74
SKIL	6.00	7.40	7.90	16.0	20.4	28.7	5.20	6.20	8.60	3.90	4.40	4.60	2.50	3.00	3.50
EureKa3!	0.85	0.94	1.03	2.45	2.47	3.73	1.29	0.94	1.9	0.69	0.66	0.75	0.52	0.53	0.69

*Reported values are absolute amplitude in microvolts (μv)

a reduction in signal amplitude which can be corrected by a scaling factor (Ferree, 2000). Additionally, different windowing methods affect the signal amplitude in slightly different ways (Smith, 1997). Although the corrective factors are not specified, SKIL uses a 75% overlap of a Hanning Window, EureKa3! uses both Blackman and Hanning Windows, and NeuroRep's windowing is achieved by means of a first difference pre-whitening filter and a two-stage Butterworth band pass filter.

The differences between reported spectral amplitudes for each of the three programs are not a primary concern because each program's database is based on its individual spectral calculations. Where the user does need to use caution is in attempting to equate the spectral report from one program to that of another when attempting to identify the actual absolute signal amplitude for a given frequency or bandpass (e.g., calculating ratio measures).

EXPERIMENT 2

Method

Participants. The clinical sample consisted of 10 adults with ADHD (6 males and 4 females), ranging in age from 21 to 47 years, who were enrolled in undergraduate or graduate courses at a large southeastern university. Informed consent was obtained following the university's institutional review board guidelines and inclusion criteria required that each participant be formally registered with the university's Office of Disability Services with a diagnosis of ADD or ADHD. Participants were also required to demonstrate clear characteristics of the disorder as measured by personal endorsement of at least six of nine hyperactive-impulsive items, or at least six of nine inattentive symptoms, as indicated from diagnostic criteria on a DSM-IV symptom checklist for ADHD.

The control sample consisted of 10 adults aged 21-44 years (5 males and 5 females). Participants for the control group were recruited from undergraduate and graduate classes via posted flyers and class announcements. Inclusion criteria required individuals to be free of current or past history of ADHD symptomatology as assessed though the personal interview, self-report, and the *DSM-IV* symptom checklist for ADHD.

Exclusion criteria for both groups included: (a) a standard score less than 85 on the Peabody Picture Vocabulary Test–3rd Ed. (PPVT-III); (b) a history of neurological or psychiatric disorder, head injury, or substance abuse; and (c) previous diagnosis of specific learning disabilities, as assessed though an individually administered health history questionnaire and structured personal interview. To control for medication effects, ADHD participants being treated with stimulant medication were evaluated after a medication-free period of at least 12 hours. Control subjects were required to be abstinent of any type of medication except for oral contraceptives.

Electroencephalograph (EEG) Recording. EEG recordings were made using a fitted electrode cap (Electro Cap Inc.) with electrodes in an array corresponding to the International 10-20 Placement System (Jasper, 1958) referenced to linked ears. Standardized preparation involved all electrode impedances being maintained at or below 5 KOhms. There were additional electrodes placed at the outer canthus of each eye to monitor horizontal eye movement and an electrode above and below the left eye to monitor vertical eye movement. Accordingly, data from these guard channels was used during data review to aid in the elimination of epochs containing artifactual data stemming from muscle activity.

The raw EEG was collected using a Lexicor NeuroSearch-24C electroencephalograph with analog to digital converter, using version 1.51 of the NeuroLex acquisition software. Acquisitions were made with a band-pass filter set at 0.5-32 Hz, high-pass filter set to "off," and a sampling rate of 128 samples per second. The Fast Fourier Transform (FFT) utilized a Hanning window and cosine tapering.

Procedure. Participants were asked to report to the university's research laboratory in order to obtain informed consent, completion of the screening measures, and EEG recordings, with all tasks completed in a single, two-hour appointment. All data collection was performed between the hours of 8 a.m. and 1 p.m.

All participants completed five QEEG recordings comprising of two baseline conditions and three task conditions. The conditions of interest to the present study included a three-minute eyes-closed resting baseline followed by a three-minute eyes-open resting baseline. The order of administration remained standard for all participants.

The eyes-closed baseline required the participant to sit for three minutes, while remaining as motionless as possible. During the three-minute eyes-open baseline, participants were asked to gaze at a blank 17-inch computer monitor, adjusted to eye-level, approximately three feet in front of them, and were again asked to refrain from any extraneous body or eye movement.

Initial Data Analysis. The EEG data from the eyes-closed and eyes-open resting baselines was initially inspected off-line with a Pentium 200 processor using Lexicor NeuroLex software (Lexicor Medical Technology, 1992). With a sampling rate of 128 samples per second, standardized application of NeuroLex allowed the visual review of two-second epochs for gross artifact contamination with the option of accepting or rejecting entire epochs for analysis. Data from the aforementioned artifact channels was carried throughout the visual analysis to aid in differentiating phenomena attributed to the cerebral EEG and phenomena of non-cerebral origin.

The data files for the ADHD subjects were then imported into the EEG Editor (Congedo, 2001) EEG data review and editing package for additional review and artifact rejection. With the ability to select contaminated segments shorter than the epoch length (two seconds), the EEG Editor afforded additional control of data selection and artifact rejection as opposed to whole-epoch rejection. The data files for the control subjects were not subjected to any additional artifact review.

Participant data files for the eyes-closed and eyes-open resting baselines were submitted to the NeuroRep QEEG Analysis and Report System (Hudspeth, 2000) and the SKIL Topometric Software packages (Sterman & Kaiser, 2000). Only eyes-closed data was submitted to the EureKa3! QEEG Analysis Package (Congedo, 2002a) as an eyes-open database is not currently available for this package. Individual analyses and database comparisons were then generated for each program following established guidelines from their respective manuals with one exception. The exception being that no additional artifact rejection was performed with any of the three packages to ensure that identical data files were being evaluated.

Database Comparisons

NeuroRep Analyses. The NeuroRep program yielded raw and Adult QEEG Reference Database (AQRD) comparisons for four-band (Delta = 0.5-3.5 Hz; Theta = 3.5-7 Hz; Alpha = 7-13 Hz; Beta = 13-22 Hz) absolute amplitude, relative power, and relative power frequency ratios (Delta/Beta, Theta/Beta, Delta/Alpha, and Alpha/Beta), for each of the 19 channels. It also provided 171-pair wise connection maps for coherence, phase, and asymmetry for each of the four bands. Four-band Neuroelectric Images (NEIs) were also generated based on principal components analysis of cross-correlation and coherence measurements. Additional analyses provided by the NeuroRep system included single-band weighted-average maps, single-band topographies for absolute amplitude and relative power, and maps indicating single-channel FFTs and coefficients of variation (CVs) for each of the nineteen channels.

The NeuroRep AQRD database is comprised of 31 individuals for eyes-closed comparisons and 30 individuals for eyes-open comparisons; approximately 95% of the eyes-closed and eyes-open comparisons are matched. Both are comprised of non-clinical adults and college students, ranging from 22 to 42 years of age. Each individual completed the Luria-Nebraska Neuropsychological Battery and was required to meet standard criteria for normality. This included having a Pathognomicity T-Score below 70 and no more than three clinical scales with a T-Score over 70 (Hudspeth, 1999b). Exclusion criteria included: (a) a positive history for abnormal prenatal, perinatal, or postnatal development; (b) disorders of consciousness; (c) head injury; (d) diseases of the central nervous system; (e) history of seizures; (f) significant deviations in mental or physical development; and (g) substance abuse (Hudspeth, 1999b).

Aggregate data was produced for both eyes-closed and eyes-open resting baselines through the initial creation of a dummy header and EEG record file. Following individual analyses, raw scores from each individual analysis were exported from the respective output file, imported into a spreadsheet, and then averaged to produce the aggregate raw data. The aggregate raw data was then submitted against the database to produce group reports.

SKIL Analyses. SKIL produced both raw and time-of-day corrected spectral analyses for six clinical bands (Delta = 1-4 Hz; Theta = 4-8 Hz; Alpha = 8-12 Hz; SMR = 12-15 Hz; Beta1 = 15-18 Hz; Beta2 = 18-24 Hz), six-band and user-defined topometric analyses (single-state and state comparison), six-band and user-defined topographic maps, and comodulation analyses for user-defined band passes. Data were also evaluated for percentage change across eyes-closed and eyes-open states and compared with the normative database for state modulation. Finally, topographic maps displaying comodulation between all sites at the subject's dominant frequency for a given condition was compared with the normative database. All SKIL normative database comparisons for individual data comparisons were conducted with time-of-day correction enabled.

The SKIL normative database was derived from 135 individuals, ranging from 18 to 55 years of age. Approximately 80% were male and 20% female. The group consisted of students and laboratory personnel (50%), volunteers recruited from the community (25%), and U.S. Air Force personnel (25%). All were screened for significant medical history, drug use, and recent life events (Kaiser & Sterman, 2000).

The SKIL program is the only one of the three that includes a method for creating aggregate data. This is achieved through the use of its replication function. In this manner, each individual spectral result can be analyzed individually or combined with others to obtain a single average. Following the individual analyses, aggregate data were examined by enabling each individual's spectral result to produce a single average for each respective condition (eyes-closed, eyes-open).

EureKa3! Analyses. EureKa3! functions both as a stand-alone QEEG analysis package and produces data files that can be viewed with the LORETA-Key software package (Pascual-Marqui, 1999; Pascual-Marqui, Michel, & Lehmann, 1994). LORETA is the acronym for Low Resolution Electromagnetic Tomography, one of the currently available methods for addressing the EEG inverse problem. EureKa3! produced band-defined QEEG spectral amplitude and power results, peak frequency, pair-wise coherence, LORETA power, and LORETA relative power analyses. Additionally, database comparisons were produced for QEEG power, QEEG relative power and power ratios, LORETA power, and LORETA relative power and power ratios.

The EureKa3! NTE Adult Database 2A used in the current study is comprised of 84 individuals ranging from 18 to 30 years of age (M = 21.1, SD = 2.8). Thirty one of the individuals were male, 53 were female. Sixty-eight were right-handed while 16 were left handed (Congedo, 2002a). All individuals were required to have negative medical and clinical histories and a negative history for substance use within the previous 31 days. All data was collected between the hours of 11 a.m. and 2 p.m., Monday through Friday, under standardized conditions and setting (L. Sherlin, personal communication, February 26, 2003).

Aggregate EureKa3! analyses were achieved by averaging the individual results of the EureKa3! analyses. Specifically, after each individual's data file was submitted for analysis, the individual's sample proportions for each target variable were imported into a spread sheet where they were compiled and averaged. Following compilation, the average sample proportions for each target variable were examined.

Results

The clinical sample consisted of 10 adults previously diagnosed with ADHD (6 males and 4 females), aged 21-47 years (M = 29.40, SD = 7.47). These individuals yielded an aggregate estimate of intelligence in the average range (85-115) as obtained by the PPVT-III (M = 107.20, SD = 10.33, Range = 88-125). The control sample consisted of 10 non-clinical adults (5 females and 5 males) aged 21-44 years (M = 26.8, SD = 7.52). These individuals also yielded an aggregate estimate of intelligence in the average range (85-115) as obtained by the PPVT-III (M = 107.9, SD = 12.46, Range = 88-132).

The NeuroRep, SKIL, and EureKa3! packages provided unique analyses. As such, results from each package will initially be presented and then the respective results will be discussed. Results will be presented for individual subjects, aggregate group data, and for non-clinical controls.

NeuroRep

Individual Analyses. Initially, the 19-channel average peak frequency and relative power spectra reports were examined for both the eyes-closed and eyes-open conditions to identify the relative dominant frequency. The coefficient of variation for each channel's spectra was also examined to ensure quality of data. In general, a low coefficient of variation across the spectral range suggests homogeneous data and quality artifact rejection.

For the eyes-closed condition, all but one subject's dominant frequency appeared to fall within the alpha range; the one exception fell within the theta range. Six of the 10 appeared to have eyes-closed dominant frequencies below 10 Hz, or in the low-alpha (8-10 Hz) range; the other three had an eyes-closed dominant frequency in the high-alpha (10-12 Hz) range. For the eyes-open condition, 8 out of the 10 individuals had dominant frequencies in the low-alpha range; two were in the high-alpha (10-12 Hz) range. Overall, the majority of the ADHD individuals appeared to exhibit a dominant frequency within the low-alpha range for both eyes-closed and eyes-open conditions. For most of the subjects, the dominant frequency most often extended from the occipital regions to the frontocentral areas (F3, Fz, F4).

The absolute single-band magnitude topographies were then examined for overall organization. As with the relative power spectra, these most often revealed dominant activity within the 9-10 Hz range which extended from the occipital regions to frontocentral (F3, Fz, F4) regions (see Figure 1). The weighted average reference maps were also examined at this time to investigate the possibility that the apparent "frontocentral alpha" was being caused by contamination of the reference channels. The weighted average reference reduces the possibility of widespread activity contaminating the reference of all channels (Fisch, 1999; Lemos & Fisch, 1991). The NeuroRep weighted average reference maps revealed that the dominant frequency activity did in fact often extend into central regions (see Figure 1) and at times, into frontocentral (F3, Fz, F4) areas.

The relative power single-band z-score topographies were examined next. In general, as compared to the database, most of the adults with ADHD (70%) exhibited a prevalence of 7-10 Hz activity, often in central and frontal regions. Four of the 10 also exhibited activity in this range during the eyes-open baseline. Only two of the subjects displayed excesses of 5-7 Hz activity in central and frontal regions. To date, one of the more common findings in ADHD, especially in the children's literature, is increased theta, often accompanied by decreased beta activity (Lazzaro et al., 1998; Mann et al., 1992; Monastra et al., 2001; Monastra et al., 1999). However, this decrease in beta, relative to a non-clinical population, appears to lessen with age (Bresnahan et al., 1999; Bresnahan & Barry, 2002; Lubar & Lubar, 1999).

The four-band coherence and phase maps were examined for any pattern of deviation. For the eyes-closed condition, 60% of the individuals expressed a deviation from the database for at least one pair-wise connection in beta (13-22 Hz) coherence, 50% for alpha (7-13 Hz), 40% for theta (3.5-7 Hz), and 20% for delta (0.5-3.5 Hz). For the eyes-open comparison, 70% evidenced a significant deviation from the database for at least one pair-wise connection in beta coherence, 60% for alpha, and 20% for both alpha and theta. For the two conditions combined, 65% evidenced beta coherence abnormalities and 55% evidenced alpha coherence abnormalities. Although a single pattern of coherence deviations wasn't found, frontal areas appeared to be implicated most often with hypercoherences found. Frontal alpha hypercoherences were also present for several of the individuals.

With regard to phase, deviation from the database was present in all individuals, for all bands, except one individual in the alpha band. The most prevalent pattern of deviation for all ten of the individuals during the eyes-closed baseline and for eight of the ten during the eyes-open baseline was at least one right frontal (F2-Fz, Fz-F4, Fz-F8, F4-F8) hypophase relationship in the beta band. More so, in all observations

FIGURE 1. NeuroRep single-band absolute magnitude topographies and weighted average map for 21 yr male with ADHD during eyes-open baseline. Note predominance of 9-10 Hz activity despite eyes-open condition.

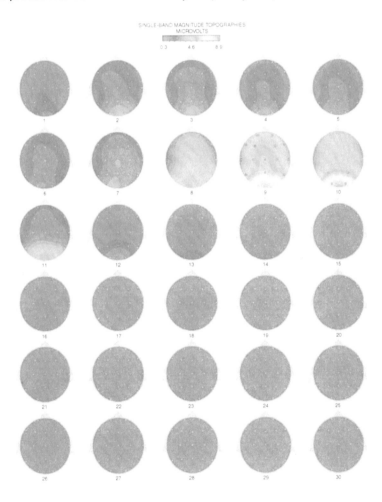

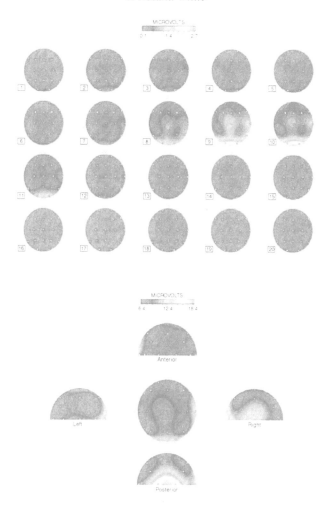

except two, this was accompanied by an increased phase relationship at F3-Fz (see Figure 2). Other phase abnormalities were observed but this pattern was characteristic for 90% (18 of the 20) possible eyes-closed and eyes-open database comparisons.

Group Analyses. Aggregate NeuroRep Adult QEEG Reference Database reports, spectral reports, and Neuroelectric Images (NEI) were generated for the 10 individuals with ADHD. As compared with the database, the group data revealed a right frontal hypophase relationship in theta, alpha, and beta, accompanied by a left frontocentral hyperphase relationship in beta for the eyes-closed condition (see Figure 3). Similar

FIGURE 2. NeuroRep coherence and phase maps for 21 yr male with ADHD during eyes-open baseline. Note frontal hypercoherence and right frontal hypophase in beta band.

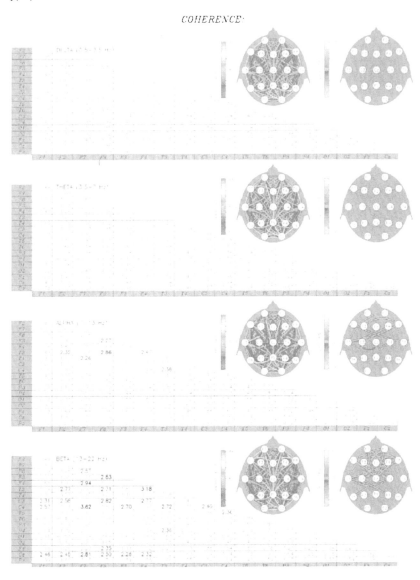

PHASE

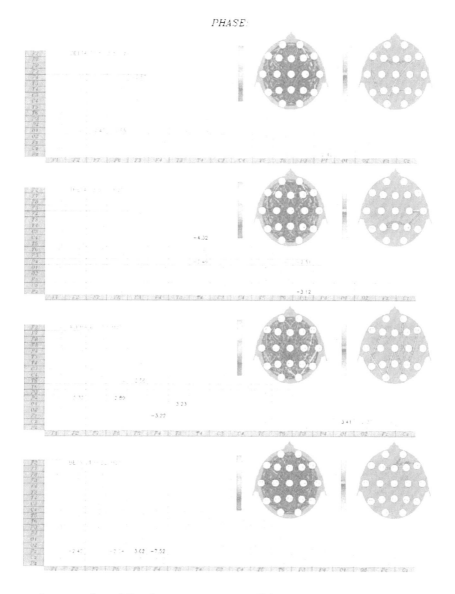

results were found for the eyes-open condition. The group data revealed no significant findings for coherence as compared against the database for either eyes-closed or eyes-open baselines.

Group spectral results indicated that 9-10 Hz activity was predominant in both conditions, as indicated by the single-band and percent

FIGURE 3. NeuroRep coherence and phase group maps for all ten adults with ADHD during eyes-closed baseline. Note right frontal hypophase in theta, alpha, and beta bands accompanied by left frontocentral hyperphase in alpha and beta.

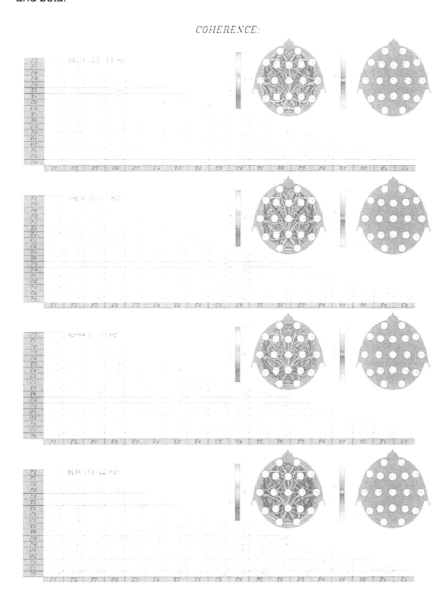

PHASE:

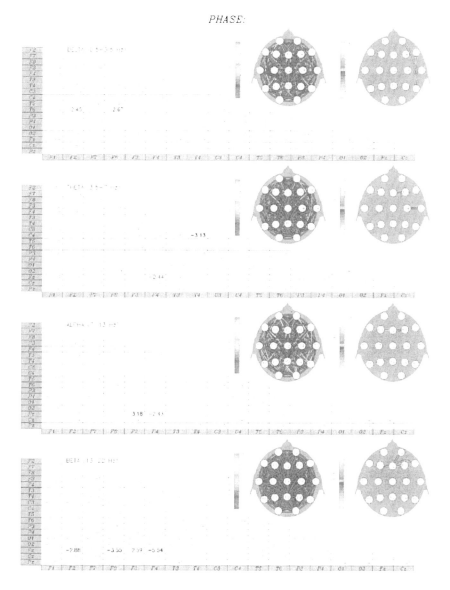

power topographies. As compared with the database, the ADHD group evidenced elevated 7-9 Hz activity in frontal areas during the eyes-closed condition and elevated 8-9 Hz activity in the same areas during the eyes-open baseline. Both conditions were characterized by slight reductions in 11-30 Hz activity in frontal areas.

With regard to absolute amplitude, the aggregate AQRD report indicated that these individuals demonstrated absolute amplitude levels that were significantly lower in various areas, across all four bands in the eyes-closed condition and in the delta, theta, and beta bands for the eyes-open condition (see Figure 4). The single-band relative power z-score maps indicated dominant activity in the 7-9 Hz range for the eyes-closed condition and dominant activity in the 8-9 Hz range for the eyes-open condition (see Figure 5). Excessive activity in the 2-3 Hz range was also present in both conditions.

The remaining aggregate results, the Neuroelectric images (NEI), suggested frontal hypercoherence in the alpha and beta bands, especially in the eyes-closed condition (see Figure 6). Furthermore, there appeared to hypocoherence between frontal and non-central posterior regions in the alpha band. It should be noted that these images are based on within-subject analyses, not database comparisons.

Analysis of Controls. Lastly, given the apparent prevalence of the right frontal hypophase in these ADHD subjects and the dominant activity within the 8-10 Hz range for both eyes-closed and eyes-open baselines, the data files from the non-clinical controls were analyzed to ensure that these findings were indeed unique to the adults with ADHD. Of the original 10 control subjects, data recordings for one subject were contaminated by a bad electrode, thus resulting in nine remaining individuals available for analysis.

NeuroRep AQRD reports were examined for each of the nine controls. All nine subjects had at least one component of the right frontal hypophase, left frontocentral hyperphase relationships as reported for the ADHD subjects. To ensure that the prevalence of the right anterior hypophase finding was not attributable to an error in data collection or acquisition device failure, three additional controls from a separate study, collected on the same acquisition device as the one used in the current investigation, and three additional ADHD subjects, whose data was collected on a different acquisition device, were also evaluated with NeuroRep. All resulted in the same right frontal hypophase findings. Therefore, the current right anterior hypophase results can be attributed to the NeuroRep Phase analysis itself, not to the ADHD group.

The AQRD coherence analyses revealed a predominance of hypercoherence findings in the beta band (8 of the 9) but the pattern of deviations was different from that of the ADHD group. Whereas the ADHD group often exhibited frontal hypercoherence, findings in the control group tended to involve the temporal electrodes, suggesting artifact contamination.

The AQRD absolute amplitude reports revealed that the control subjects also evidenced significantly lower amplitude values as compared with the database. However, inspection of these reports and the percent power topographies revealed that the controls did not exhibit the same pattern of activity as the ADHD group. Specifically, the controls demonstrated alpha predominantly in the posterior regions and exhibited attenuation of alpha during the eyes-open baseline.

The NEI's were also examined for the control group. As found for the ADHD subjects, there appeared to be increased coherence in the frontal areas in both the alpha and the beta bands. However, the apparent anterior-posterior disconnect in alpha coherence was not present for these individuals.

As with the ADHD group, aggregate reports were also generated. For the control groups' data, there were two deviations from the database in beta coherence: increased coherence between Cz and T5 for the eyes-closed condition and increased coherence between F3 and T5 in the eyes-open condition. The apparent right frontal hypophase relationship was present in the eyes-closed condition for the control groups' data but not in the eyes-open group map.

There were low absolute amplitudes in all bands, across most areas of the scalp, according to the z-score absolute amplitude table and map. Relative delta was also below normative levels for both conditions. The control group also demonstrated alpha attenuation during the eyes-open condition as compared to the eyes-closed condition.

The control groups' aggregate NEI suggested increased frontal coherence in the alpha and beta bands, but not to the extent as was suggested with the ADHD group. Furthermore, the apparent anterior-posterior hypocoherence seen in the ADHD group was not present for the control group.

SKIL

Individual Analyses. Foremost, each ADHD subject's spectral data for the six pre-defined clinical bands was examined as compared with the normative database, with time-of-day correction, in grid view. For the eyes-closed condition, all subjects demonstrated elevated spectral amplitudes for the Delta (1-4 Hz), Beta1 (15-18 Hz), and Beta2 (18-24 Hz) bands. Seventy percent demonstrated elevated theta (4-8 Hz), 90% demonstrated elevated alpha (8-12 Hz), and 60% demonstrated elevated SMR (12-15 Hz) at C3, Cz, or C4.

FIGURE 4. NeuroRep absolute amplitude group z-score maps for all ten adults with ADHD during eyes-closed and eyes-open baselines.

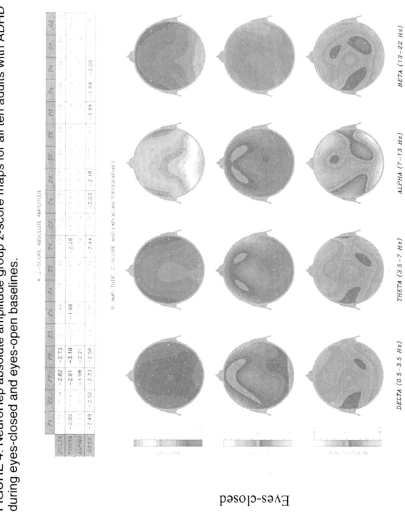

Eyes-closed

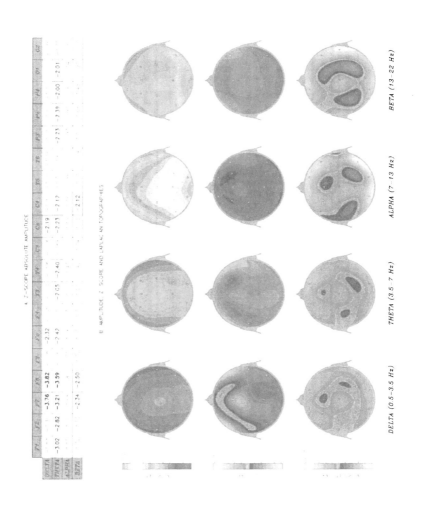

Eyes-open

145

FIGURE 5. NeuroRep single-band relative power z-score group maps for all ten adults with ADHD during eyes-closed and eyes-open baselines. Note predominance of 7-9 Hz activity in the eyes-closed condition and predominance of 8-9 Hz activity in the eyes-open condition.

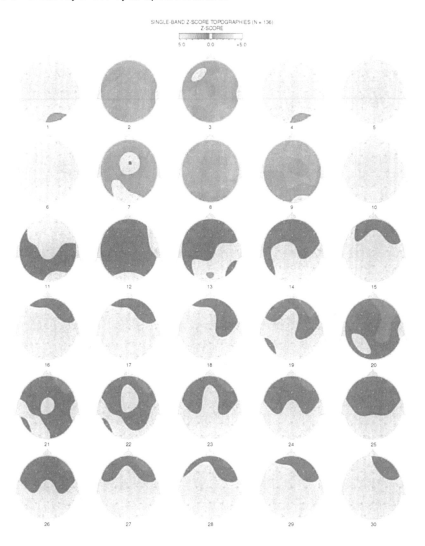

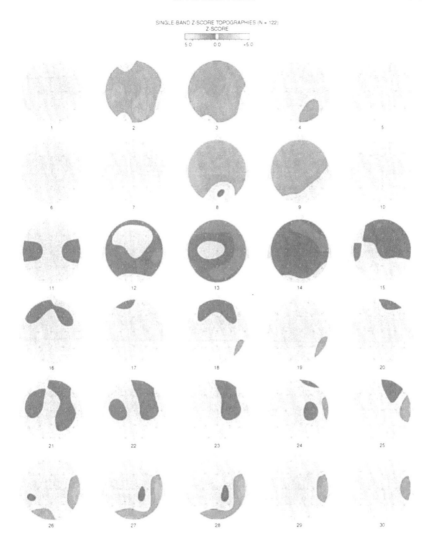

For the eyes-open condition, 100% of the subjects demonstrated elevated delta and beta2 as compared with the database. Furthermore, 80% had elevated theta, 60% had elevated alpha, 60% had elevated SMR (at C3, Cz, or C4), and 80% had elevated beta1 activity. Overall, most subjects demonstrated elevated spectral values as compared with the database for all bands and most scalp locations. The elevated delta was expected because the SKIL user's manual recommends that data be col-

FIGURE 6. NREP neuroelectric images for ADHD aggregate eyes-closed baseline data. Note proximity of frontal electrodes in alpha and beta coherence in horizontal view and apparent distances in alpha in the sagittal view. The uppermost images are anatomical references.

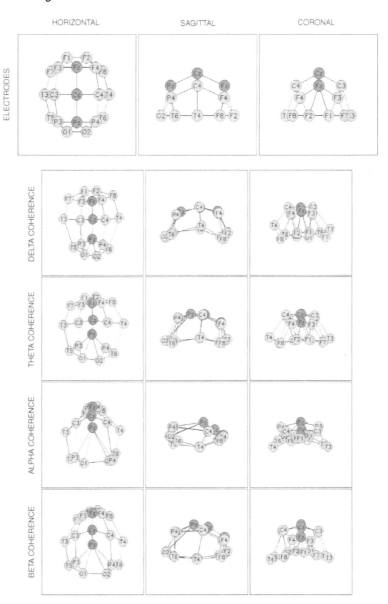

lected with a 2 Hz high-pass filter engaged. The data collection for the current sample did not employ such a filter.

After examining the spectral values in grid view, database comparisons were then examined in topometric view. As indicated in examination of the spectral grids, subjects tended to demonstrate elevated spectral amplitudes across bands and locations (see Figure 7). These findings support previous research that found adults with ADHD have significantly higher levels of absolute power activity across the spectral band as compared to controls (Bresnahan & Barry, 2002).

The spectral data for each individual was also examined for percentage change across eyes-closed and eyes-open baselines. Only three individuals demonstrated significant changes as compared against the database (two for alpha; two for SMR, beta1, and beta2). As previously indicated, these individuals demonstrated elevated levels in both conditions.

Each subject's topographic display was examined for both clinical-band and single Hz activity. This revealed that these ADHD adults demonstrated dominant activity generally within the 8-10 Hz range for both eyes-closed and eyes-open baselines. Each individual's dominant frequency was then used for the comodulation analyses. In general, these adults typically displayed an apparent hypercomodulation in frontal areas (70% of eyes-closed; 60% of eyes-open) or an apparent frontal-posterior disconnect (see Figures 8 and 9).

Group Analyses. Group maps were then generated for the SKIL analyses. Absolute amplitude topographies are displayed in Figure 10 for the six clinical bands. Statistical maps for the same data indicated significant elevations in all bands across the entire scalp. The aggregate comodulation map was examined next. Although not as robust as some of the individual cases, the group data suggested frontal hypercomodulation in the average dominant frequency (9-10 Hz) during both eyes-closed and eyes-open resting baselines, but it was more prevalent during the eyes-closed condition (see Figure 11). When the group comodulation data was compared against the database, a slight frontal-posterior disconnect appears to be present, but as in the raw comodulation group data, it is less robust for the overall group (see Figure 11).

Analysis of Controls. The nine non-clinical controls were evaluated in the same manner as the group analysis. For the eyes-closed condition, the absolute amplitude topographies and topometric displays indicated significantly elevated levels of delta across the scalp and significantly

FIGURE 7. SKIL topometric display of database comparisons for 24 yr female with ADHD during eyes-open baseline. Results are shown for the delta, theta, alpha, and beta1 bands.

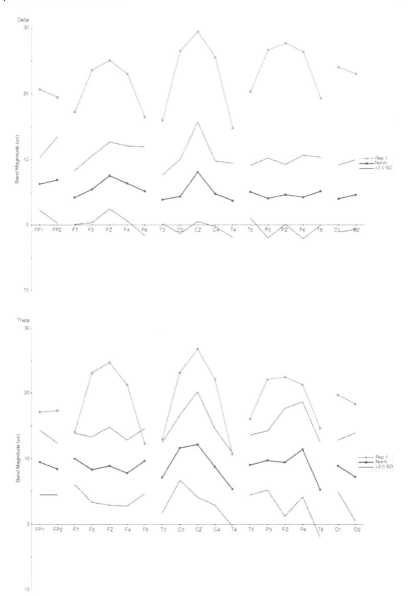

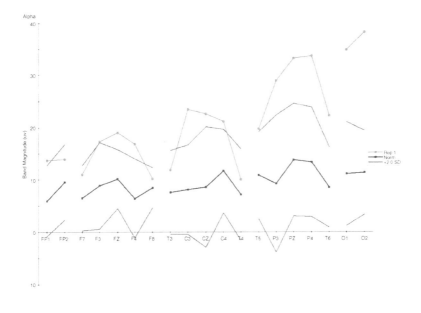

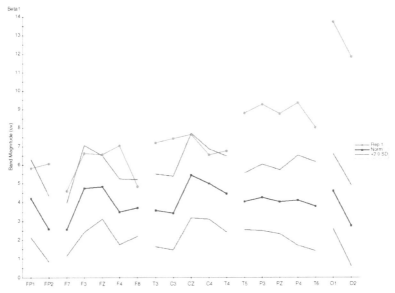

FIGURE 8. SKIL single-band topographies (top) and both raw (bottom left) and database comparison (bottom right) comodulation maps for 21 yr male with ADHD during eyes-closed baseline. Note frontal hypercomodulation at dominant frequency (9-10 Hz) accompanied by apparent frontal-posterior disconnection.

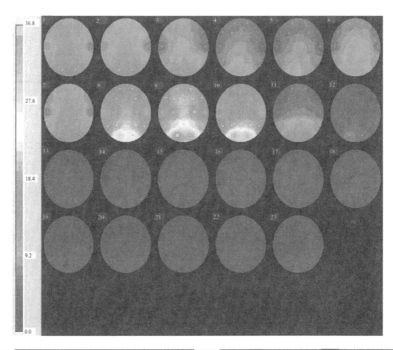

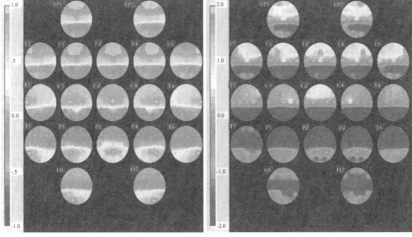

FIGURE 9. SKIL single-band topographies (top) and both raw (bottom left) and database comparison (bottom right) comodulation maps for 21 yr male with ADHD during eyes-open baseline. Note predominance of 9-10 Hz activity despite eyes-open condition and corresponding frontal hypercomodulation at dominant frequency.

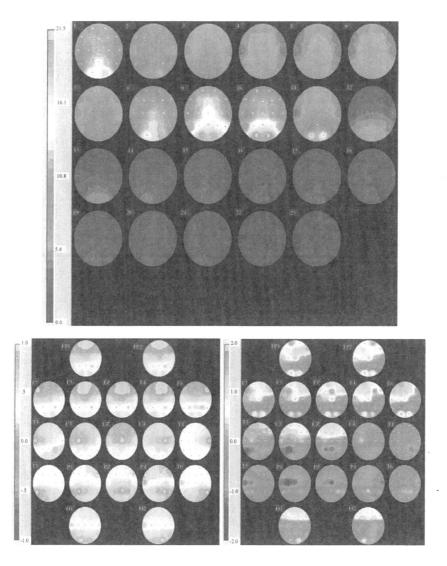

FIGURE 10. SKIL clinical-band topographies for group aggregate eyes-closed (top) and eyes-open (bottom) baselines. Note predominance of alpha activity during both conditions.

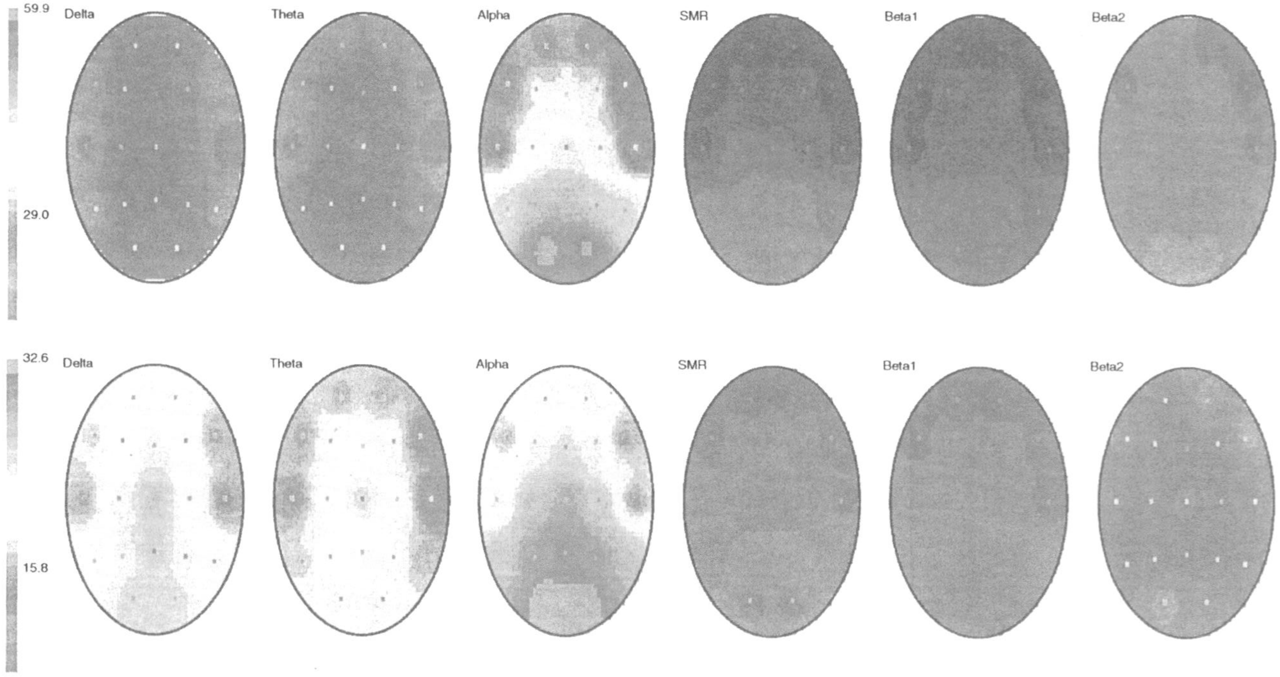

FIGURE 11. SKIL raw and database comparison comodulation maps for ADHD aggregate eyes-closed and eyes-open baselines at dominant frequency (9-10 Hz). Note frontal hypercomodulation in the raw data (top) and apparent frontal-posterior disconnect in the statistical (bottom) comparisons, especially for the eyes-closed condition.

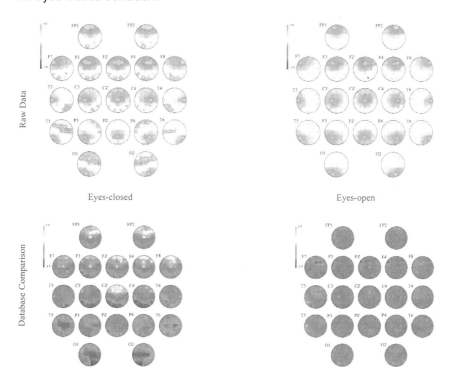

higher frontal theta. Both alpha and SMR were within normal limits while significantly increased levels of beta1 and beta2 were reported.

For the eyes-open condition, the same displays indicated significantly elevated levels of delta and theta across the scalp. Alpha and SMR were again within normal limits. Five central and posterior sites had elevated beta1 and 14 sites had elevated beta2.

The dominant rhythm for the controls' eyes-closed baseline appeared to be within the 9-11 Hz range. The group comodulation maps for both the raw group data and statistical comparison were negative for any apparent hyper- or hypocomodulation. The control groups' dominant rhythm for the eyes-open baseline appeared to be in the 6-8 Hz range; again both raw and statistical evaluations of comodulation data failed to produce any significant results.

EureKa3!

Individual Analyses. Currently, EureKa3! only has an eyes-closed database available for data comparisons. Hence, only eyes-closed comparisons will be reported for this package. Additionally, three of the subjects were excluded from the current analyses due to being beyond the age limits of the database, resulting in seven individuals being evaluated with this package.

After submitting the remaining seven eyes-closed data files to EureKa3! for analysis, the respective analysis report or worksheet was examined. This report summarizes both the QEEG and LORETA database comparisons for absolute power, relative power, and power ratios.

For absolute QEEG power, two of the seven individuals with ADHD differed significantly from the database. One individual had lower levels of activity in the delta (2-3.5 Hz) and theta (4-7.5 Hz), and low frequency (2-7.5 Hz) bands at frontal and central sites; the other had elevated levels of alpha1 (8-10 Hz) activity at frontal and central sites. Five individuals did not have any significant absolute QEEG power findings for their eyes-closed baselines.

For relative QEEG power, three individuals had significant deviations from the database. Two individuals had significantly higher levels of alpha (8-12 Hz) or alpha1 activity accompanied by significantly lower levels of beta (13-21 Hz) activity over the entire scalp. The other individual had lower levels of relative theta and low-frequency activity at T5. Four individuals did not have any significant relative QEEG power findings for their eyes-closed baselines.

It should be noted that EureKa3! reports significance levels for not only univariate comparisons, but also provides an additional analysis, the Deviancy Test (Congedo, 2002a), to account for multiple comparisons. Thus, it is possible for a finding to be significant at the univariate level but to be insignificant after accounting for multiple comparisons. In fact, of the four individuals that did not have significant QEEG power findings overall, all four had significant univariate comparisons, but these findings were not maintained after accounting for multiple comparisons.

The comparisons for LORETA absolute power were examined next. All seven demonstrated significance variations at the univariate level but only two had significant findings that were maintained after accounting for multiple comparisons. One individual demonstrated lower absolute delta and theta current source density in BA 36, the fusiform gyrus. The other had lower absolute beta current source density in BA

11, the left orbitofrontal gyrus, an area that has been found to be significantly smaller in a recent magnetic resonance volumetry study of adults ($n = 8$) with ADHD (Hesslinger et al., 2002).

The relative LORETA power analyses revealed that all seven individuals had at least one significant finding at the univariate level but only two maintained significant deviations after accounting for multiple comparisons. One individual had significantly lower levels of relative theta current source density in BA 20, the left inferior temporal gyrus. The other individual demonstrated increased levels of alpha in BA 36, the right fusiform gyrus, and increased alpha1 in BA 20, the left inferior temporal gyrus, accompanied by lower levels of beta1 in BA 11, the left rectal gyrus (posterior orbitofrontal gyrus; see Figure 12).

Lastly, the individual spectral amplitude files were examined with the EureKa3! Chart Editor. This application includes a module for identifying the dominant frequency for a given spectral amplitude file. These adults with ADHD demonstrated a dominant frequency within the low-alpha band ($M = 9.70$, $SD = 0.39$) for their eyes-closed baseline. Examination of the spectral amplitude files also indicated that activity within this band was not limited to occipital areas and most often extended into central and frontal regions.

Group Analyses. As with the NeuroRep and SKIL analyses, group data were generated from the EureKa3! analyses. Specifically, group data was averaged to create LORETA relative power database comparisons, absolute QEEG power, and relative QEEG power database comparisons.

With regard to the aggregate QEEG data, there were no significant deviations from the database for either absolute or relative power. However, the highest levels were found for alpha and alpha1 activity. For the 13 bands of relative LORETA power, none met statistical significance for the aggregate data as compared against the EureKa3! database.

Analysis of Controls. Seven of the 10 controls were evaluated with EureKa3!; two were excluded due to the age range of the database, and a third was excluded due to having a bad channel in the data record. Four of the seven had at least one significant finding as compared to the database after accounting for multiple comparisons. Three individuals demonstrated significantly lower levels of absolute theta current source density (two at BA 20–inferior temporal gyrus; one at BA 18–inferior occipital gyrus). The two that had significantly lower theta current source density in BA 20 also had significantly lower levels of total absolute current source density in BA 11, the posterior orbitofrontal

FIGURE 12. Significant LORETA relative power maps for 28 yr male with ADHD during eyes-closed baseline. Intersection of black arrows indicates location of maximum relative power in the respective band. Red indicates higher levels as compared to the database whereas blue signifies lower levels as compared to the database.

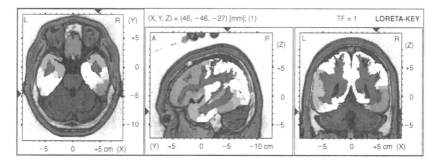

Relative Alpha (8-12.5 Hz)

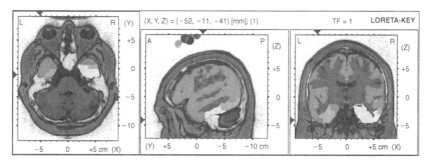

Relative Alpha1 (8-10 Hz)

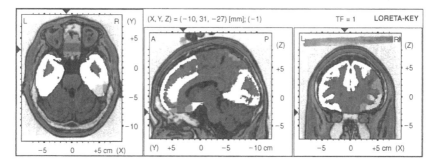

Relative Beta 1 (12-16 Hz)

gyrus. This area was implicated in the ADHD subjects but for lower beta activity.

The one individual that had excessive activity as compared to the database yielded elevated levels of relative QEEG scalp activity in the beta3 and beta4 bands and relative current source density in the high frequency, beta3, and beta4 bands in BA 20, the inferior temporal gyrus. It would be difficult to attribute this finding to any other phenomena other than residual artifact. It should be noted that LORETA analyses are extremely sensitive to artifact and the data files for the controls were not subjected to additional artifact review after gross review with the acquisition software.

With regard to spectral amplitudes, the controls' eyes-closed baseline revealed a dominant frequency within the high-alpha band (M = 10.50, SD = 0.82). This activity was most often present in the occipital and parietal channels.

Discussion

Overall, analyses provided by the three programs appear to offer potential markers for this group of adults with ADHD. The most prevalent and common finding between the three programs was a predominance of activity within the 8-10 Hz range for both eyes-closed and eyes-open conditions. Otherwise stated, there was an absence of normal alpha attenuation during the eyes-open baseline as compared with the eyes-closed baseline. Furthermore, this activity often extended into central and frontal regions, beyond the typical occipital and parietal regions.

Another common finding appears to be decreased level of cortical differentiation in frontal areas as evidenced by the frontal hypercomodulation findings in SKIL and the Neuroelectric (NEI) images in NeuroRep. The NEI findings were most evident in the alpha bandpass whereas the SKIL hypercomodulation was evident for the individual's dominant frequency, which most often fell within the same bandpass (specifically 8-10 Hz). These two analyses also suggested reduced communication between anterior and posterior regions, again for activity within the alpha band as revealed by the SKIL statistical comodulation display and the NeuroRep NEI for alpha coherence. These findings suggest at least partial congruence between the two programs for apparent alterations in cortical functional connectivity.

There were mixed results for spectral amplitude. The NeuroRep results indicated significantly lower levels of absolute delta, theta, and beta whereas SKIL indicated significantly higher absolute values across the spectral range. The eyes-closed comparison against the EureKa3! database did not indicate any consistent amplitude differences when accounting for multiple comparisons but there was indication of elevated relative alpha1 (8-10 Hz) in both the univariate QEEG and LORETA analyses.

Some apparently significant results were not supported when the control subjects were evaluated. The most striking was the apparent reduction in phase values involving right frontal regions for the ADHD group as reported by the NeuroRep AQRD database comparison. Further investigation revealed that almost every data file evaluated had these same findings.

EXPERIMENT 3

Method

Given the apparent differences observed during Experiments 1 and 2 between the three programs, it seemed necessary to compare the three programs with regard to percent power calculations. This third experiment was performed by calculating and comparing percent power for 1-23 Hz activity, as reported by all three packages, for the ADHD subjects' aggregate eyes-closed baseline data. This analysis was examined in the effort to determine if the aforementioned discrepant results were due to inherent differences between each database or if the programs differed in the manner in which they calculate spectral amplitude, which would in turn be reflected in percent power calculations.

Procedure. Single-band spectral amplitudes for each of the 19 channels, as reported from each program, were imported into MS Excel where they were first squared to obtain absolute power and then summed accordingly to produce five non-overlapping spectral bins (1-4 Hz, 5-7 Hz, 8-12 Hz, 13-18 Hz, and 19-23 Hz). The total power for a given site was then calculated by summing the spectral bin values. Each spectral bin's power for a given channel was then divided by the channel's total power, resulting in the respective spectral bin's percent power value for that site.

Results

The results are displayed in Table 3. Although similar, the percent power results were not entirely congruent across the different band

TABLE 3. Calculated Percent Power for Aggregate ADHD Eyes-Closed Baselines

NeuroRep

	FP1	FP2	F7	F3	FZ	F4	F8	T3	C3	CZ	C4	T4	T5	P3	PZ	P4	T6	O1	O2
1-4 Hz	15.4	15.4	15.6	14.1	14.0	14.0	14.7	12.6	12.6	13.6	12.6	12.5	8.8	9.5	10.3	10.2	8.5	7.9	8.1
5-7 Hz	12.3	12.5	12.2	13.4	13.7	13.3	11.7	11.0	12.0	12.7	12.2	10.4	7.9	8.6	9.2	8.8	7.9	5.8	5.9
8-12 Hz	53.2	54.3	50.3	53.8	54.9	54.8	53.1	49.4	56.7	56.5	56.7	48.9	64.0	64.3	64.2	63.3	65.7	70.2	69.9
13-18 Hz	12.6	12.0	14.4	12.4	11.7	12.2	13.6	18.0	12.5	11.5	12.7	18.2	13.6	12.4	11.7	12.6	12.8	11.4	11.4
19-23 Hz	6.5	5.8	7.5	6.2	5.6	5.8	6.8	9.1	6.2	5.7	5.9	10.0	5.7	5.1	4.6	5.0	5.0	4.8	4.6

SKIL

	FP1	FP2	F7	F3	FZ	F4	F8	T3	C3	CZ	C4	T4	T5	P3	PZ	P4	T6	O1	O2
1-4 Hz	33.4	34.1	33.3	27.9	27.1	28.0	33.1	26.0	25.2	26.5	25.7	27.1	17.9	19.9	21.7	21.6	17.5	16.1	16.7
5-7 Hz	10.3	10.2	10.4	12.1	12.4	12.0	10.1	10.2	11.1	11.8	11.5	10.0	7.9	8.5	9.1	8.7	7.8	6.1	6.2
8-12 Hz	42.8	43.1	40.6	45.9	47.3	46.5	42.2	42.8	48.8	48.2	48.4	41.7	58.5	57.5	56.2	55.8	60.2	64.8	64.0
13-18 Hz	9.1	8.8	10.8	9.7	9.1	9.4	10.0	14.4	10.4	9.4	10.1	14.3	11.4	10.3	9.6	10.3	10.6	9.5	9.6
19-23 Hz	4.4	3.8	4.9	4.4	4.1	4.1	4.5	6.5	4.6	4.1	4.2	6.9	4.2	3.8	3.4	3.6	3.9	3.5	3.5

EureKa3!

	FP1	FP2	F7	F3	FZ	F4	F8	T3	C3	CZ	C4	T4	T5	P3	PZ	P4	T6	O1	O2
1-4 Hz	28.8	29.6	31.4	19.8	18.9	19.3	30.9	22.9	18.2	22.7	18.1	21.5	13.7	15.3	19.1	16.3	13.0	13.6	13.3
5-7 Hz	8.6	8.7	8.8	9.0	9.0	8.6	9.4	9.5	9.4	10.4	9.6	10.3	7.4	7.3	8.1	7.4	7.9	6.0	6.0
8-12 Hz	49.1	49.0	44.1	55.8	58.9	57.2	44.1	44.7	54.1	52.6	54.0	44.8	63.0	62.0	59.1	60.8	63.8	67.7	67.8
13-18 Hz	9.2	8.8	10.7	10.5	9.1	10.2	10.8	15.9	11.9	9.4	12.2	15.9	11.8	11.3	10.2	11.3	11.5	9.4	9.6
19-23 Hz	4.3	3.9	4.9	4.9	4.2	4.6	4.8	7.1	6.4	4.9	6.1	7.5	4.2	4.2	3.5	4.1	3.8	3.3	3.2

passes and varied slightly across bandpasses and different areas of the scalp. See Table 4 for a list of differences between the minimum and maximum values recorded for each bandpass and for each site. The differences range from a maximum of 18.68% between SKIL and NeuroRep for the 1-4 Hz bin to a 0.10% difference between the three programs for a single site in the 5-7 Hz bin.

Discussion

Regardless of possible differences in reported amplitude values, it would seem that the three packages would approach congruence with

TABLE 4. Differences Between Minimum and Maximum Percent Power Values Calculated for the Three Programs

	1-4 Hz	5-7 Hz	8-12 Hz	13-18 Hz	19-23 Hz
FP1	17.94	3.72	10.39	3.42	2.21
FP2	18.68	3.85	11.20	3.22	1.91
F7	17.72	3.35	9.74	3.73	2.60
F3	13.72	4.45	9.93	2.72	1.80
FZ	13.09	4.70	11.63	2.66	1.58
F4	14.02	4.68	10.75	2.75	1.65
F8	18.38	2.31	10.92	3.63	2.25
T3	13.45	1.51	6.59	3.55	2.56
C3	12.57	2.64	7.88	2.16	1.87
CZ	12.88	2.27	8.29	2.11	1.57
C4	13.13	2.58	8.28	2.55	1.92
T4	14.64	0.46	7.12	3.91	3.15
T5	9.10	0.57	5.45	2.14	1.58
P3	10.41	1.38	6.86	2.10	1.37
PZ	11.43	1.16	7.96	2.12	1.19
P4	11.44	1.38	7.58	2.28	1.42
T6	8.95	0.10	5.46	2.22	1.23
O1	8.16	0.30	5.34	2.02	1.44
O2	8.57	0.23	5.88	1.77	1.40

regard to percent power if similar algorithms were being used by each. It appears that the three programs in fact differ to some extent in their basic spectral analyses. Furthermore, the programs vary according to bandpass and channel, which may be due to different FFT, windowing, and smoothing parameters used by the three programs.

OVERALL SUMMARY AND CONCLUSIONS

Foremost, it should be noted that the intended purpose of the present investigation was not to suggest that database "A" is better than database "B" or database "B" is better than database "C." The aim of the current investigation was to examine and compare the respective results of three currently available databases for a given clinical population. Thus, the current investigation sought to potentially identify unique or common markers for this particular clinical group when using each of the respective database packages.

Another primary point that must be made concerns the small sample sizes examined in this study and the number of comparisons that were made in both individual and aggregate formats. Although every effort was made to maintain experimental rigor, the current results can not be widely attributed to the adult ADHD population as a whole. The current study should be used as a preliminary investigation or source of debate for future investigations of adult ADHD and QEEG or QEEG databases.

This investigation examined a sample of adults previously diagnosed with Attention Deficit Hyperactivity Disorder (ADHD) and their respective comparisons against three of the currently available QEEG reference databases (NeuroRep v4, SKIL v2.05, and EureKa3!). By using subjects with an *a priori* diagnosis, both individual and aggregate results could be examined for this diagnostic category. Given the seeming paucity of QEEG data for adults with ADHD, it was uncertain what results would be revealed. As such, it seemed necessary to first compare the three programs with data of known parameters.

When files were analyzed that consisted of a 10 Hz, 20 µv peak amplitude sinusoidal signal, all three programs produced different results. Only the results of the NeuroRep analysis produced spectral amplitude values that approached the original 20 µv signal (see Table 1). When the programs were compared with a data file from a single control subject, again there were differences in absolute spectral amplitudes but it appeared that NeuroRep and EureKa3! produced similar results whereas

SKIL's values were generally higher. These results have at least one important implication. Namely, the apparent inability to verify or directly compare an individual's spectral amplitude values between programs.

Following the preliminary analysis of the signal files, the data for the adult ADHD subjects was analyzed with each package. In addition to focusing on group homogeneity, data homogeneity was also a concern. As such, the exact same data files for each individual's eyes-closed and eyes-open baselines were submitted to each package (only the eyes-closed baseline was submitted to EureKa3!). This was accomplished through the incorporation of an independent program for data review and artifact rejection, the EEG Editor (Congedo, 2001).

Typically, unless all artifact review is performed with a researcher's or clinician's acquisition software, the data editors within each package are used. All three analysis packages offer advanced data editors. However, despite the increased control over artifact review afforded by each, at the time of this study, neither NeuroRep nor SKIL allow the artifact-rejected data file to be exported for use in other packages. Therefore, unless a professional only uses their acquisition and review software for artifact review, or an independent editor capable of exporting the artifact-rejected file, apparent differences between packages could possibly be attributed to slightly different data files actually being subjected for analysis.

Each of the packages appeared to offer possible QEEG markers for adult ADHD but not all potential markers held up to additional scrutiny. For example, the results of the NeuroRep analysis suggested right frontal phase deviations in the beta band (13-22 Hz). These database deviations were in the negative direction, suggesting a decreased phase relationship or reduced transmission time between right frontal sites. This finding seemed congruent with the current neuroimaging literature of ADHD and frontal involvement (Amen & Carmichael, 1997; Benson, 1991; Grodzinsky & Barkley, 1999; Johnson et al., 2001; Lovejoy et al., 1999), and specifically findings of right frontal involvement in ADHD (Casey et al., 1997; Castellanos et al., 1996).

However, in an effort to ensure that this potential marker was indeed unique for adults with ADHD, the same analysis was performed for nine non-clinical controls. Their results also indicated right frontal hypophase relationships in the beta band. As an additional step, three additional controls from a separate study, collected on the same acquisition device as the one used in the present study, and three additional ADHD subjects, whose data was collected on a different acquisition device, were also examined. All showed the same right frontal hypophase findings. Hence, this is apparently a characteristic of the NeuroRep AQRD Phase analysis, and not a characteristic unique to adult ADHD.

Features suggested by NeuroRep that did appear to be unique to the ADHD group were predominance of 8-10 Hz activity in the eyes-closed condition and predominance of 7-10 Hz activity in the eyes-open condition. Absolute spectral amplitudes were depressed for both ADHD and controls. The NeuroRep Neuroelectric Images (NEIs) suggested frontal hypercoherence in the alpha and beta bands and an apparent hypo-coherence in the alpha band between anterior and posterior regions. The NEI is not based on a database comparison and is a within-subject analysis. This finding was interesting in that the coherence analysis for the aggregate ADHD data failed to find any significant deviations in coherence as compared with the database.

However, besides the small sample size, it is possible that the individual patterns of coherence deviation were suppressed in the aggregate data. In fact, a recent investigation of working memory using positron emission tomography (PET) revealed that adults with ADHD failed to demonstrate a consistent pattern of regional cerebral blood flow (rCBF) change related to the completion of a working memory task (Schweitzer et al., 2000). In contrast, non-clinical controls completing the same task tended to demonstrate rCBF changes in similar cortical areas (Schweitzer et al., 2000). Although each individual in the clinical group had a diagnosis of ADHD, it is possible that there are different patterns of cortical anomalies associated with this diagnosis, just as it has been demonstrated in children (Barry et al., 2003). This finding also affects other comparisons in the current study, especially given the small sample size.

Results of the SKIL analysis suggested frontal hypercomodulation and increased spectral amplitudes for the ADHD group. The elevated spectral amplitudes is supportive of previous research suggesting that adults with ADHD generally demonstrate higher levels of absolute power across the spectral range (Bresnahan & Barry, 2002). The SKIL analysis also suggested a predominance of 8-10 Hz activity for both eyes-closed and eyes-open conditions.

Combined, the results of the individual NeuroRep coherence and NEI analyses and the apparent hypercomodulation revealed by the SKIL analysis suggest a lack of cortical differentiation in frontal areas for this group of adults with ADHD. The EureKa3! LORETA analysis also revealed some indication of frontal lobe involvement. These findings appear to support previous studies that have implicated frontal lobe dysfunction in individuals with ADHD (Amen & Carmichael, 1997;

Benson, 1991; Casey et al., 1997; Castellanos et al., 1996; Grodzinsky & Barkley, 1999; Hesslinger et al., 2002; Johnson et al., 2001; Lovejoy et al., 1999).

The apparent prevalence of alpha activity for these individuals has several implications in light of recent findings associated with this range of EEG activity. Traditionally, alpha has been viewed as a rhythm that most often appears during relaxed wakefulness, usually with the eyes-closed, which is attenuated with eyes-opening, attention, or mental activity (Fisch, 1999; Niedermeyer, 1999). Contemporary research has produced results that are incompatible with the concept of alpha reflecting cortical idling.

A recent investigation into the role of alpha activity revealed that mean alpha amplitude was higher in internally-directed attention as opposed to externally-directed attention (Cooper, Croft, Dominey, Burgess, & Gruzelier, 2003). Other studies have also suggested that the lower alpha band reflects attentional processes whereas the upper alpha band is implicated in semantic memory processes (Klimesch, 1997). These findings have direct implications for the current results. While one component of ADHD is inattention to external stimuli, subjective reports by several of the adult ADHD subjects in the current study suggest instead that their personal experience of ADHD is characterized by increased attention to internal foci. The current sample also demonstrated elevated levels of low-alpha activity during both eyes-closed and eyes-open baselines. Taken in conjunction, the elevated low-alpha activity demonstrated by these subjects would appear to be supportive of increased alpha during internally-directed attentional states as suggested by the Cooper et al. (2003) study.

Lastly, as compared to the other two packages, the EureKa3! analyses seemingly did not appear to offer as many potential QEEG markers for this particular group of adults with ADHD. There was support for increased levels of activity in the 8-10 Hz range but few other consistent findings for the individuals analyzed. However, it is important to note that EureKa3! is the only package of the three that actively addresses the issue of multiple comparisons and the possibility of "significant" findings by chance alone, or Type I errors. While it is possible that the number of findings for the other two packages could possibly be attributed to chance when the total number of possible comparisons is calculated, it is quite likely that the apparently fewer number of "significant" findings with EureKa3! can be attributed to a more conservative approach to data analysis. This possibility of a Type II error is further impacted when evaluating group QEEG data that has the potential for heterogeneity if you examine the children's literature (Barry et al., 2003; Chabot & Serfontein, 1996; Clarke et al., 2001). Studies comprised of larger sample sizes, and attention to the issue of multiple comparisons, are needed to fully address these issues.

In conclusion, it appears that QEEG reference databases may prove useful in the evaluation of adult ADHD. They appear to offer information as to how an individual compares against a normative group that may not be available otherwise. They also offer analyses that may not otherwise be readily available. However, until such time that there is a greater convergence of results between such programs, or a clearer indication of specific divergence, it will be difficult to fully ascertain their true potential for clinical or research applications with adult ADHD.

REFERENCES

Amen, D. G., & Carmichael, B. D. (1997). High-resolution brain SPECT imaging in ADHD. *Annals of Clinical Psychiatry, 9* (2), 81-86.

Barry, R. J., Clarke, A. R., & Johnstone, S. J. (2003). A review of electrophysiology in attention-deficit/hyperactivity disorder: I. Qualitative and quantitative electroencephalography. *Clinical Neurophysiology, 114* (2), 171-183.

Benson, D. F. (1991). The role of frontal dysfunction in attention deficit hyperactivity disorder. *Journal of Child Neurology, 6* (Suppl.), S9-S12.

Bresnahan, S. M., Anderson, J. W., & Barry, R. J. (1999). Age-related changes in quantitative EEG in attention-deficit/hyperactivity disorder. *Biological Psychiatry, 46* (12), 1690-1697.

Bresnahan, S. M., & Barry, R. J. (2002). Specificity of quantitative EEG analysis in adults with attention deficit hyperactivity disorder. *Psychiatry Research, 112* (2), 133-144.

Casey, B. J., Castellanos, F. X., Giedd, J. N., Marsh, W. L., Hamburger, S. D., Schubert, A. B. et al. (1997). Implication of right frontostriatal circuitry in response inhibition and attention-deficit/hyperactivity disorder. *Journal of the American Academy of Child and Adolescent Psychiatry, 36* (3), 374-383.

Castellanos, F. X., Giedd, J. N., Marsh, W. L., Hamburger, S. D., Vaituzis, A. C., Dickstein, D. P. et al. (1996). Quantitative brain magnetic resonance imaging in attention-deficit hyperactivity disorder. *Archives of General Psychiatry, 53* (7), 607-616.

Chabot, R. J., & Serfontein, G. (1996). Quantitative electroencephalographic profiles of children with attention deficit disorder. *Biological Psychiatry, 40* (10), 951-963.

Clarke, A. R., Barry, R. J., McCarthy, R., & Selikowitz, M. (1998). EEG analysis in Attention-Deficit/Hyperactivity Disorder: A comparative study of two subtypes. *Psychiatry Research, 81* (1), 19-29.

Clarke, A. R., Barry, R. J., McCarthy, R., & Selikowitz, M. (2001). EEG-defined subtypes of children with attention-deficit/hyperactivity disorder. *Clinical Neurophysiology, 112* (11), 2098-2105.

Congedo, M. (2001). EEG Editor (Version 2.0) [Computer software]. Knoxville, TN: Nova Tech EEG, Inc.

Congedo, M. (2002a). EureKa! (Version 3.0) [Computer software]. Knoxville, TN: NovaTech EEG, Inc.

Congedo, M. (2002b). WaveGeneratore [Computer software]. Knoxville, TN: NovaTech EEG, Inc. [available at http://www.novatecheeg.com]

Cooper, N. R., Croft, R. J., Dominey, S. J. J., Burgess, A. P., & Gruzelier, J. H. (2003). Paradox lost? Exploring the role of alpha oscillations during externally vs. internally directed attention and the implications for idling and inhibition hypotheses. *International Journal of Psychophysiology, 47* (1), 65-74.

Ferree, T. C. (2000). *EGI technical note: Inferring signal amplitudes from discrete (FFT) power values.* Electrical Geodesics, Inc. Retrieved January 18, 2003 from: www. ftp://ftp.egi.com/pub/documentation/technotes/SignalAmplitude.pdf

Fisch, B. J. (1999). *Fisch and Spehlmann's EEG primer: Basic principles of digital and analog EEG* (3rd ed.). New York: Elsevier.

Grodzinsky, G. M., & Barkley, R. A. (1999). Predictive power of frontal lobe tests in the diagnosis of Attention Deficit Hyperactivity Disorder. *The Clinical Neuropsychologist, 13* (1), 12-21.

Hesslinger, B., Tebartz van Elst, L., Thiel, T., Haegele, K., Hennig, J., & Ebert, D. (2002). Frontoorbital volume reductions in adult patients with attention deficit hyperactivity disorder. *Neuroscience Letters, 328* (3), 319-321.

Hudspeth, W. J. (1999a). NeuroRep QEEG Analysis and Report System (Version 4.0) [Computer software]. Reno, Nevada: Gray Matter, Inc.

Hudspeth, W. J. (1999b). NeuroRep: The QEEG analysis and report system–User's guide (Version 4.0). Reno, Nevada: Gray Matter, Inc.

Jasper, H. H. (1958). The ten twenty electrode system of the international federation. *Electroencephalography and Clinical Neurophysiology, 10*, 371-375.

Johnson, D. E., Epstein, J. N., Waid, L. R., Latham, P. K., Voronin, K. E., & Anton, R. F. (2001). Neuropsychological performance deficits in adults with attention deficit/hyperactivity disorder. *Archives of Clinical Neuropsychology, 16* (6), 587-604.

Kaiser, D. A., & Sterman, M. B. (2000). *SKIL topometric software manual.* Retrieved October 25, 2000 from: http://www.skiltopo.com/manual.htm

Klimesch, W. (1997). EEG-alpha rhythms and memory processes. *International Journal of Psychophysiology, 26* (1-3), 319-340.

Lazzaro, I., Gordon, E., Whitmont, S., Plahn, M., Li, W., Clarke, S. et al. (1998). Quantified EEG activity in adolescent attention deficit hyperactivity disorder. *Clinical Electroencephalography, 29* (1), 37-42.

Lemos, M. S., & Fisch, B. J. (1991). The weighted average reference montage. *Electroencephalography and Clinical Neurophysiology, 79* (5), 361-370.

Lexicor Medical Technology (1992). NeuroLex™ Software for EEG–Data Acquisition & Analysis (Version 1.51) [Computer software]. Boulder, CO: Lexicor Medical Technology.

Lovejoy, D. W., Ball, J. D., Keats, M., Stutts, M. L., Spain, E. H., Janda, L. et al. (1999). Neuropsychological performance of adults with attention deficit hyperactivity disorder (ADHD): Diagnostic classification estimates for measures of frontal lobe/executive functioning. *Journal of the International Neuropsychological Society, 5*, 222-233.

Lubar, J. F., & Lubar, J. O. (1999). Neurofeedback assessment and treatment for attention deficit/hyperactivity disorders. In J. R. Evans & A. Abarbanel (Eds.), *Introduction to quantitative EEG and neurofeedback* (pp. 103-143). San Diego: Academic Press.

Mann, C. A., Lubar, J. F., Zimmerman, A. W., Miller, C. A., & Muenchen, R. A. (1992). Quantitative analysis of EEG in boys with attention-deficit-hyperactivity disorder: Controlled study with clinical implications. *Pediatric Neurology, 8* (1), 30-36.

Monastra, V. J., Lubar, J. F., & Linden, M. (2001). The development of a quantitative electroencephalographic scanning process for Attention Deficit-Hyperactivity Disorder: Reliability and validity studies. *Neuropsychology, 15* (1), 136-144.

Monastra, V. J., Lubar, J. F., Linden, M., VanDeusen, P., Green, G., Wing, W. et al. (1999). Assessing attention deficit hyperactivity disorder via quantitative electroencephalography: An initial validation study. *Neuropsychology, 13* (3), 424-433.

Niedermeyer, E. (1999). The normal EEG of the waking adult. In E. Niedermeyer & F. H. Lopes da Silva (Eds.), *Electroencephalography: Basic principles, clinical applications, and related fields* (4th ed., pp. 149-173). Baltimore: Williams & Wilkins.

Pascual-Marqui, R. D. (1999). Review of methods for solving the EEG inverse problem. *International Journal of Bioelectromagnetism, 1* (1), 75-86.

Pascual-Marqui, R. D., Michel, C. M., & Lehmann, D. (1994). Low resolution electromagnetic tomography: A new method for localizing electrical activity in the brain. *International Journal of Psychophysiology, 18* (1), 49-65.

Schweitzer, J. B., Faber, T. L., Grafton, S. T., Tune, L. E., Hoffman, J. M., & Kilts, C. D. (2000). Alterations in the functional anatomy of working memory in adult attention deficit hyperactivity disorder. *American Journal of Psychiatry, 157* (2), 278-280.

Smith, S. W. (1997). *The scientist and engineer's guide to digital signal processing* (2nd ed.). San Diego: California Technical Publishing.

Sterman, M. B., & Kaiser, D. A. (2000). SKIL QEEG analysis software (Version 2.05) [Computer software]. Bel Air, CA: Sterman-Kaiser Imaging Laboratory.

White, J. N., Jr. (2001). *Neuropsychological and electrophysiological assessment of adults with attention deficit hyperactivity disorder.* Unpublished doctoral dissertation, The University of Tennessee, Knoxville.

Index

Accuracy measures, 24-27
Acquisition procedures, 60-61
ADD (attention deficit disorder), 79-80
ADHD (attention deficit hyperactivity
        disorder), 123-169
Adult ADHD (attention deficit
        hyperactivity disorder)
        evaluations
basic signal analyses and, 123-169
vs. childhood evaluations,
        123-124,135
future perspectives of, 163-167
historical perspectives of, 124-126
introduction to, xiii-xviii,123-126
QEEG (quantitative
        electroencephalographic)
        reference databases for,
        123-169
    Blackman and Hanning
        Windows and, 129-130
    eyes open vs. eyes closed
        baselines for, 128,131-163
    FFT (Fast Fourier Transform)
        and, 130-132,163
    introduction to, 123-126
    Lexicor Health Systems data
        acquisition equipment
        (NeuroSearch and NeuroLex)
        and, 123-131
    linked ear references vs. average
        references and, 127
    LORETA (Low Resolution
        Electromagnetic Tomography),
        133,156-159

NEIs (neuroelectric images) and,
        131-143,159-166
NeuroRep QEEG Analysis and
        Report System, 124-167
NovaTech EureKa3! QEEG
        Analysis System, 124-167
PET (positron emission
        tomography) and, 165
SKIL Topometric QEEG
        Software Package, 124-167
SMR (sensorimotor rhythm),
        effects of, 135-149,155
WaveGeneratore and, 126
Z-scores and, 135-146
reference and research literature
        about, 167-169
standardized measurement
        instruments for, 125-132
    DSM-IV symptom checklists,
        129
    IVA (Intermediate Visual and
        Auditory) Continuous
        Performance Test, 125
    Luria-Nebraska
        Neuropsychological Battery,
        132
    PPVT-III (Peabody Picture
        Vocabulary Test-3rd Ed.), 130
    WCST (Wisconsin Card Sorting
        Test), 125
studies of, 126-163
    experiment 1, 126-129
    experiment 2, 129-160
    experiment 3, 160-163

Adult QEEG Reference Database,
NeuroRep. *See* NeuroRep
QEEG Analysis and Report
System
American Psychiatric Association. *See*
APA (American Psychiatric
Association)
Amplifiers and digital matching, 99
Anterior-posterior sequential
placements, 39
APA (American Psychiatric
Association), 57,65
AQRD (Adult QEEG Reference
Database), NeuroRep. *See*
NeuroRep QEEG Analysis
and Report System
Artifacts
data of, 40-42
rejection techniques for, 63
removal of, 96-97
Attention deficit disorder. *See* ADD
(Attention deficit disorder)
Attention deficit hyperactivity
disorder, adult. *See* Adult
ADHD (attention deficit
hyperactivity disorder)
evaluations
Average references, 97,127

Baselines, eyes open vs. eyes closed,
128,131-163
Basic signal analyses, 123-169
BEAM (brain electrical activity
mapping), 48
Biofeedback applications. *See* Clinical
neurotherapy (biofeedback)
applications
Biver, C. J., 87-121
Blackman and Hanning Windows,
129-130
Brain electrical activity mapping. *See*
BEAM (brain electrical
activity mapping)
Brain mapping, 69-76

Channel numbers, 61-62
Childhood ADHD (attention deficit
hyperactivity disorder)
evaluations, 123-124,135
Clinical neurotherapy (biofeedback)
applications
brain mapping, 69-76
FFT (Fast Fourier Transform)
and, 71-74
introduction to, 69-70,74
multi-channel recording
analyses and, 75-76
ethical considerations of, 81-83
homeostasis and, 82
iatrogenesis and, 82
introduction to, 81
neurological-psychological
integrations and, 81-82
future perspectives of, 82-83
introduction to, xiii-xviii,69-70
neurofeedback, 69-70
historical perspectives of, 70-71
introduction to, 69-70
protocols for, 71
SMR (sensorimotor rhythm)
and, 70-71
in neurophysiology, 71-72
EEG (electroencephalography)
techniques, 71-72
International Federation of
Clinical Neurophysiology
and, 72
introduction to, 71
normative databases for, 76-79
disadvantages of, 79
importance of, 76-77
introduction to, 76-77
normality assessments and,
77-78
proposal for, 81-82
protocols for, 71,79-80
ADD (attention deficit disorder)
and, 79-80
epilepsy and, 79
introduction to, 71,79

SMR (sensorimotor rhythm)
and, 79-80
reference and research literature
about, 83-85
spectral analyses, 72-74
Comparison criteria sets
for associated tests, 60
benefits of, 55
in clinical settings, 56
criticism of, 65-66
electrophysiological procedures
and, 60-65
acquisition procedures and,
60-61
artifact rejection techniques and,
63
channel numbers and, 61-62
confounding variables and, 63
introduction to, 60-61
linked ear references and, 60-61
montages and, 60-61
recording procedures and, 62
screening techniques and, 64-65
statistical methods and, 65
task conditioning and, 64
time-of-day effects and, 63-64
EOG (ElectroOculogram) leads, use
of, 62
future perspectives of, 54,65-66
historical perspectives of, 54-56
of Hudspeth, W. J., 57-58,61-65
introduction to, xiii-xviii,48,53-56
of John, E. R., 57-65
lack of, 53
reference and research literature
about, 67-68
reliability of, 55-56
for specific databases, 57-65
LSNDB/NeuroGuide (Thatcher
Lifespan Normative EEG
Database), 57,59-65
neurometric analysis systems,
57-59,61-65
NeuroRep QEEG Analysis and
Report System, 57-59,61-65

SKIL Topometric QEEG
Software Package, 57,59-65
standardized measurement
instruments and, 60
McCarthy Intelligence Scale, 60
Vineland Social Maturity Scale,
60
WIPPSI (Wechsler Intelligence
Preschool and Primary Scale
of Intelligence), 60
of Sterman, M. B. and Kaiser, D.
A., 57-65
surveys of, 53-68
introduction to, 53-56
methods, 56-65
normality criteria, 57-58
participants, 57-58
results, 65-66
of Thatcher, R. W., 57-65
uses of, 54-56
Complex demodulation computations,
97-98
Congedo, M., 1-29
Construction and use of comparison
databases
databases, definition of, 33-34
discriminant analyses and, 32,48-49
FFT (Fast Fourier Transform) and,
32
future perspectives of, 50
introduction to, xiii-xviii, 31-33
montage reformatting and, 37-40
correct vs. best, 38-39
G1 (grid one) vs. G2 (grid two)
and, 37-39
global averaging and, 40
Hjorth derivations and, 38-40
Laplacian technique and, 38-40
linked ear references and, 38-40
minimum guidelines for, 39
selection of, 40
sequential placements
(anterior-posterior and
transverse), 39
varieties of, 39-40

visualized vs. localized spikes,
    38-40
MRI (magnetic resonance imaging)
    and, 33-34
normative reference comparisons
    and, 33-37
    definition of, 31
    derived features and, 36
    of EEG (electroencephalography)
        features, 34-37
    EPs (evoked potentials) vs.
        ERPs (event-related
        potentials), 36
    introduction to, 33-34
    linked ear references and, 37
    mean values vs. standard
        deviations, 35-36
    normalcy and, 33-34
    norming and, 34-37
    P300 components and, 37
    pattern deviation evaluations,
        34-35
    spectral power measures, 35-36
pediatric, 34
PET (positron emission
    tomography) and, 34
in practice, 42-48
    BEAM (brain electrical activity
        mapping), 48
    comparisons of, 48,53-68
    International Brain Database,
        45-47
    introduction to, 42
    LORETA (Low Resolution
        Electromagnetic
        Tomography), 47
    LSNDB/NeuroGuide (Thatcher
        Lifespan Normative EEG
        Database), 43-44,48-49
    neurometrics and, 42-49
    NeuroRep QEEG Analysis and
        Report System, 47
    SKIL Topometric QEEG
        Software Package, 44-45

reference and research literature
    about, 50-52
surveys of, 31-52
validation and, 40-42
    artifact data and, 40-42
    deviations and, 41-42
    introduction to, 40
    non-medication supplements and
        agents, 41
Criteria sets, comparison. *See*
        Comparison criteria sets
Cross-validation, 100-103
Curtin, R., 87-121

Databases, definition of, 33-34
Daubert factors, 88-89,101-102,106
Demodulation computations, complex,
    97-98
Dickson, P., 53-68
Digital matching and amplifiers, 99
Discriminant analyses, 32,48-49
DSM-IV symptom checklists, 129
Duffy, F. H., 48

ElectroOculogram leads. *See* EOG
    (ElectroOculogram) leads
Electrophysiological procedures, 60-65
EOG (ElectroOculogram) leads, 62
Epilepsy, 79
EPs (evoked potentials) vs. ERPs
    (event-related potentials), 36
Ethical considerations, 81-82
EureKa3!. *See* NovaTech EureKa3!
    QEEG Analysis System
Event-related potentials. *See* EPs
    (evoked potentials) vs. ERPs
    (event-related potentials)
Evoked potentials. *See* EPs (evoked
    potentials) vs. ERPs
    (event-related potentials)
Eyes open vs. eyes closed baselines,
    128,131-163

Fast Fourier Transform. *See* FFT (Fast Fourier Transform)
FFT (Fast Fourier Transform), 2-3, 25-26,32,71-74,97-98,103, 130-132,163
Future perspectives
  of adult ADHD (attention deficit hyperactivity disorder) evaluations, 163-167
  of clinical neurotherapy (biofeedback) applications, 82-83
  of comparison criteria sets, 54
  of construction and use of comparison databases, 50
  of PM (parametric) vs. nPM (non-parametric) accuracy comparisons, 24-27
  of validation and clinical correlations, 119

Gaussian distributions
  vs. non-gaussian, 9-12
  vs. normal, 99-100
Global averaging, 40
Gunkelman, J., 31-52

Historical perspectives
  of Adult ADHD (attention deficit hyperactivity disorder) evaluations, 124-126
  of comparison criteria sets, 54-56
  of neurofeedback, 70-71
  of PM (parametric) vs. nPM (non-parametric) accuracy comparisons, 2-3
Hjorth derivations, 38-40
Homeostasis, 82
Hudspeth, W. J., 47-58,61-65

Iatrogenesis, 82
Images, neuroelectric. *See* NEIs (neuroelectric images)

Instruments, standardized. *See* Standardized measurement instruments
Integrations, neurological-psychological, 81-82
Intermediate Visual and Auditory Continuous Performance Test. *See* IVA (Intermediate Visual and Auditory) Continuous Performance Test
International Brain Database
  Brain Resource Company and, 46
  introduction to, 45-46
  MRI (magnetic resonance imaging) and, 47
  P300 components and, 47
  tests of, 46-47
    psychological test battery, 46-47
    psychophysiology paradigms, 47
International Federation of Clinical Neurophysiology, 72
IVA (Intermediate Visual and Auditory) Continuous Performance Test, 125

John, E. R., 42-65
Johnstone, J., 31-52

Kaiser, D. A., 57-65
Kurtosis vs. skewness, 9-13,25-27, 99-100

Left-handed vs. right-handed tests, 13-15,19-23
Lexicor Health Systems data acquisition equipment (NeuroSearch and NeuroLex), 123-131,151
Lifespan EEG reference database, 93
Linked ear references, 37-40,60-61, 98-99,127
Localized vs. visualized spikes, 38-40

Lorensen, T. D., 53-68
LORETA (Low Resolution
    Electromagnetic Tomography),
    133,156-159
    Adult ADHD (attention deficit
        hyperactivity disorder)
        evaluations and, 133,156-159
    database construction and, 47
    PM (parametric) vs. nPM
        (non-parametric) accuracy
        comparisons and, 3,9,26-27
    validation and clinical correlations
        and, 90
Low Resolution Electromagnetic
    Tomography. *See* LORETA
    (Low Resolution
    Electromagnetic
    Tomography)
LSNDB/NeuroGuide (Thatcher Lifespan
    Normative EEG Database)
    comparison criteria sets and, 57,59-65
    database construction and, 43-49
    validation and clinical correlations
        and, 88-121
Lubar, J. F., xv-xviii,1-29
Luria-Nebraska Neuropsychological
    Battery, 132

Magnetic resonance imaging. *See* MRI
    (magnetic resonance imaging)
Mapping
    BEAM (brain electrical activity
        mapping), 48
    brain. *See* Brain mapping
    SPM (Significance Probability
        Mapping). *See* SPM
        (Significance Probability
        Mapping)
McCarthy Intelligence Scale, 60,94-95
Measurement instruments, standardized.
    See Standardized measurement
    instruments
Montages and montage reformatting,
    37-40,60-61

MRI (magnetic resonance imaging),
    3,33-34
Multi-channel recording analyses,
    75-76

NEIs (neuroelectric images),
    131-143,159-166
Neuroelectric images. *See* NEIs
    (neuroelectric images)
Neurofeedback, 69-70
Neurological-psychological
    integrations, 81-82
Neurometrics, 42-49,57-65
NeuroRep QEEG Analysis and Report
    System
    Adult ADHD (attention deficit
        hyperactivity disorder)
        evaluations and, 124-167
    comparison criteria sets and, 57-65
    database construction and, 47
NeuroSearch and NeuroLex (Lexicor
    Health Systems data
    acquisition equipment),
    123,126-127,130-131
Normalcy, 33-34
Normality
    assessments of, 77-78
    criteria for, 57-58
Normative databases
    for clinical neurotherapy
        (biofeedback) applications,
        76-79
    comparisons of, 33-37
    validation and clinical correlations
        and, 88-121
Norming, 34-37
North, D. N., 87-121
NovaTech EureKa3! QEEG Analysis
    System, 47,124-167
nPM (non-parametric) accuracy
    comparisons. *See* PM
    (parametric) vs. nPM
    (non-parametric) accuracy
    comparisons

Parametric accuracy comparisons. *See*
  PM (parametric) vs. nPM
  (non-parametric) accuracy
  comparisons
Pattern deviation evaluations, 34-35
Peabody Picture Vocabulary Test-3rd
  Ed. *See* PPVT-III (Peabody
  Picture Vocabulary Test-3rd
  Ed.)
PET (positron emission tomography),
  34,165
PM (parametric) vs. nPM
  (non-parametric) accuracy
  comparisons
  accuracy measures, 24-27
    introduction to, 24
    PM (parametric) vs. nPM
    (non-parametric)
    performance and, 24-25
    SN (sensitivity), 24-27
    SP (specificity), 24-27
    TA (true acceptance), 24-27
    TR (true rejection), 24-27
  database development and, 25-27
  diagnostic systems and, 5-8
  ET (electromagnetic tomography)
    and, 2-27
    introduction to, 2-3
    LORETA (Low Resolution
    Electromagnetic
    Tomography), 3,9,26-27
    MRI (magnetic resonance
    imaging) and, 3
  FFT (Fast Fourier Transform) and,
    2-3,25-26
  future perspectives of, 24-27
  historical perspectives of, 2-3
  introduction to, xiii-xviii,1-3
  nPM (non-parametric method), 10-15
    introduction to, 13
    vs. PM (parametric method), 10
    proportions basis of, 13-15
    right-handed vs. left-handed
    tests and, 13-15
    two-tailed tests and, 15

PM (parametric method), 8-13
  gaussian vs. non-gaussian
  distributions and, 9-12
  introduction to, 8-9
  kurtosis vs. skewness and,
  9-13,25-27
  vs. nPM (non-parametric)
  method, 8,10
  SPM (Significance Probability
  Mapping) and, 9
  Z-score basis of, 8-13
reference and research literature
  about, 27-29
signal detection theory and, 5-8
  deviance probabilities, 8
  introduction to, 5-6
  inverse probabilities, 8
simulation studies of, 15-27
  alpha level manipulations for, 17
  gaussianity manipulations for, 18
  implications of, 24-27
  introduction to, 15-17
  results of, 18-23
  right-handed vs. left-handed
  tests and, 19-23
  sample size manipulations for,
  17-18
  simulation entries for, 16-17,24
Positron emission tomography. *See*
  PET (positron emission
  tomography)
Potentials, EPs (evoked potentials) vs.
  ERPs (event-related
  potentials), 36
PPVT-III (Peabody Picture Vocabulary
  Test-3rd Ed.), 130
Predictive validity, 107-112
Protocols, training, 71,79-80
Psychological-neurological
  integrations, 81-82

QEEG (quantitative
  electroencephalographic)
  analysis databases

in adult ADHD (attention deficit
        hyperactivity disorder)
        evaluations, 123-169
    clinical neurotherapy (biofeedback)
        applications for, 69-85
    comparison criteria sets for,
        48,53-68
    construction and use of, 31-52
    introduction to, xiii-xviii
    (PM) parametric vs. nPM
        (non-parametric) accuracy
        comparisons of, 1-29
    validation and clinical correlations
        of, 87-121
Quality control procedures, 96-97

Recording
    multi-channel analyses of, 75-76
    procedures for, 62
Reference and research literature
    about adult ADHD (attention deficit
        hyperactivity disorder)
        evaluations, 167-169
    about clinical neurotherapy
        (biofeedback) applications,
        83-85
    about comparison criteria sets, 67-68
    about construction and use of
        comparison databases, 50-52
    about PM (parametric) vs. nPM
        (non-parametric) accuracy
        comparisons, 27-29
    about validation and clinical
        correlations, 119-121
Reliability, comparison criteria sets,
    55-56
Right-handed vs. left-handed tests,
    13-15,19-23
Romano-Micha, J., 69-85

Scientific evidence admissibility,
    88-89,101-106
Screening techniques, 64-65

Selection criteria, 40
Sensitivity. *See* SN (sensitivity)
Sensorimotor rhythm. *See* SMR
    (sensorimotor rhythm)
Sequential placements
    (anterior-posterior and
    transverse), 39
Signal analyses, basic, 123-169
Signal detection theory, 5-8
Significance Probability Mapping. *See*
    SPM (Significance
    Probability Mapping)
Simulation studies, 15-27
Skewness vs. kurtosis, 9-13,25-27,
    99-100
SKIL Topometric QEEG Software
    Package
    Adult ADHD (attention deficit
        hyperactivity disorder)
        evaluations and, 124-167
    comparison criteria sets and, 57-65
    database construction and, 44-45
SMR (sensorimotor rhythm),
    70-80,135,147-149,155
SN (sensitivity), 24-27
SP (specificity), 24-27
Specificity. *See* SP (specificity)
Spectral analyses, 72-74
Spikes, visualized vs. localized, 38-40
SPM (Significance Probability
    Mapping), 9
Standardized measurement instruments
    DSM-IV symptom checklists, 129
    IVA (Intermediate Visual and
        Auditory) Continuous
        Performance Test, 125
    Luria-Nebraska Neuropsychological
        Battery, 132
    McCarthy Intelligence Scale,
        60,94-95
    PPVT-III (Peabody Picture
        Vocabulary Test-3rd Ed.),
        130
    Vineland Social Maturity Scale,
        60,94-95

WAIS (Wechsler Adult Intelligence
Scale), 94-95
WCST (Wisconsin Card Sorting
Test), 125
WIPPSI (Wechsler Intelligence
Preschool and Primary Scale
of Intelligence), 60,94-95
WISC-R (Wechsler Intelligence
Scale for Children), 94-95
WRAT (Wide Range School
Achievement Test), 94-95
Sterman, M. B., 57-65

TA (true acceptance), 24-27
Task conditioning, 64
Thatcher, R. W., 43-65,87-121
Time-of-day factors, 63-64,95-96
Topometric (SKIL) QEEG Software
Package. *See* SKIL Topometric
QEEG Software Package
TR (true rejection), 24-27
Training protocols, 71,79-80
Transverse sequential placements, 39
Trudeau, D. L., xiii-xiv
True acceptance. *See* TA (true
acceptance)
Two-tailed tests, 15

Use and construction of comparison
databases. *See* Construction
and use of comparison
databases

Validation and clinical correlations
database construction and, 40-42
Daubert factors, 88-89,101-106
future perspectives of, 119
introduction to, xiii-xviii,87-89
for Lifespan EEG reference
database, 93
for LORETA (Low Resolution
Electromagnetic Tomography),
90

of LSNDB/NeuroGuide (Thatcher
Lifespan Normative EEG
Database), 88-121
for normative databases, 88-121
amplifiers and digital matching
and, 99
artifact removal for, 96-97
average references for, 97
clinical correlations of, 103-107
complex demodulation
computations for, 97-98
content validity of, 112-116
cross-validation of, 100-103
current source density (CSD)
and, 97-99
demographic and gender criteria
for, 92-95
effect sizes of, 117
FFT (Fast Fourier Transform)
and, 97-98,103
gaussian vs. normal distributions
of, 99-100
inclusion and exclusion criteria,
92-94
intelligence and school
achievement criteria for,
94-95
introduction to, 88-89
kurtosis vs. skewness of, 99-100
Laplacian and, 97-99
linked ear references for, 98-99
nPM (non-parametric) methods
for, 115-118
peer reviewed vs. independent
publications and, 118-119
predictive validity of, 107-112
production of, 89-91
quality control procedures for,
96-97
recording procedures for, 96
statistical foundations of, 99-107
subject and variable selections,
91-92
time-of-day factors for, 95-96
uncontrollable factors for, 95-96

uses for, 88-89
validation steps for, 90-91
Z-scores and, 90-91,102-103,
    108-112
reference and research literature
    about, 119-121
standardized measurement
    instruments and, 94-95
    McCarthy Intelligence Scale,
        94-95
    Vineland Social Maturity Scale,
        94-95
    WAIS (Wechsler Adult
        Intelligence Scale), 94-95
    WIPPSI (Wechsler Intelligence
        Preschool and Primary Scale
        of Intelligence), 94-95
    WISC-R (Wechsler Intelligence
        Scale for Children), 94-95
    WRAT (Wide Range School
        Achievement Test), 94-95
Validity, predictive, 107-112
Vineland Social Maturity Scale,
    60,94-95
Visualized vs. localized spikes, 38-40

WAIS (Wechsler Adult Intelligence
    Scale), 94-95
Walker, R. A., 87-121
WaveGeneratore, 126
WCST (Wisconsin Card Sorting Test),
    125

Wechsler Adult Intelligence Scale. *See*
    WAIS (Wechsler Adult
    Intelligence Scale)
Wechsler Intelligence Preschool and
    Primary Scale of Intelligence.
    See WIPPSI (Wechsler
    Intelligence Preschool and
    Primary Scale of
    Intelligence)
Wechsler Intelligence Scale for
    Children. *See* WISC-R
    (Wechsler Intelligence Scale
    for Children)
White, J. N., 123-169
Wide Range School Achievement
    Test. *See* WRAT (Wide
    Range School Achievement
    Test)
WIPPSI (Wechsler Intelligence
    Preschool and Primary Scale
    of Intelligence), 60,94-95
Wisconsin Card Sorting Test. *See*
    WCST (Wisconsin Card
    Sorting Test)
WISC-R (Wechsler Intelligence Scale
    for Children), 94-95
WRAT (Wide Range School
    Achievement Test), 94-95

Z-scores, 8-13,90-91,102-103,108-112,
    135-146

Printed and bound by CPI Group (UK) Ltd, Croydon, CR0 4YY

17/10/2024

01775667-0002